CANCER
FITNESS

Exercise Programs for Cancer Patients and Survivors

Anna L. Schwartz, FNP, Ph.D., FAAN

A Fireside Book
Published by Simon & Schuster
New York   London   Toronto   Sydney

FIRESIDE
Rockefeller Center
1230 Avenue of the Americas
New York, NY 10020

For information regarding special discounts for bulk purchases,
please contact Simon & Schuster Special Sales at 1-800-456-6798
or business@simonandschuster.com

Designed by Jaime Putorti

Manufactured in the United States of America

10 9 8 7 6 5 4 3

Library of Congress Cataloging-in-Publication Data

Schwartz, Anna L.
    Cancer fitness : exercise programs for cancer patients and survivors / Anna L. Schwartz.
      p. cm.
    Includes index.
      1. Cancer—Exercise therapy. 2. Cancer—Physical therapy. I. Title.

RC271.P44S39 2004
616.99'4062—dc22   2004045340

ISBN 0-7432-3801-X

I DEDICATE THIS BOOK TO:

My patients and colleagues who have taught me so
much and made an enormous difference in my
life and work

Christine, my mother and best friend, who taught
me to reach for my dreams and follow my heart

Roberta Adams, M.D., and Saundra Buys, M.D.,
with compassion and love you held my hand
and walked me through a most challenging
chapter of life

Daniel Shapiro, who encouraged me to pursue this
book and is an inspiration to me

Betsy King, whose enthusiasm and passion for life
pushed me to accomplish more than my dreams

My dear friends Susanna Cunningham, Kathleen
Jennings, and Kerri Winters, who patiently read
and re-read drafts and provided wonderful
insight and ideas

Sabra Jones, who embodied the ideas of this book
by truly living life to the fullest, following her
dreams and making a tremendous difference in
this world for so many people. May we all have
her courage, determination and inspiration to
follow our hearts and "walk in beauty"—
hozhoni.

I would like to thank my agent, Judith Riven, for believing in
me and encouraging me to pursue this work.

DISCLAIMER

This publication contains the opinions and ideas of its author. It is intended to provide helpful and informative material on the subjects addressed in the publication. It is sold with the understanding that the author and publisher are not engaged in rendering medical, health, or any other kind of personal professional services in the book. The reader should consult his or her medical, health, or other competent professional before adopting any of the suggestions in this book or drawing inferences from it.

The author and publisher specifically disclaim all responsibility for any liability, loss, or risk, personal or otherwise, incurred as a consequence, directly or indirectly, of the use and application of any of the contents of this book.

CONTENTS

CONTENTS

FOREWORD

Exercising may be one of the best things you can do for yourself during and after your cancer treatment. Remaining active during this period was key for me in getting through metastatic testicular cancer in the best possible shape, both physically and mentally. In fact, I firmly believe that my exercise program—specially designed to accommodate my treatments and resulting change in physical ability—got me into the mental and physical condition that was necessary for me to be able to win the Tour de France. But you don't have to be a professional or even an amateur athlete to benefit from physical activity during and after your treatment. This excellent and informative guide by Dr. Anna Schwartz shows you how you can take your well-being into your own hands and do wonders for yourself. It is just the kind of empowerment that we at the Lance Armstrong Foundation strive to provide to people living with, through, and beyond cancer. From her personal experience as a cancer survivor and oncology nurse, and years of study, Dr. Schwartz offers knowledge and guidance that allows you to be instrumental in ensuring your own improved quality of life during and following cancer. Cancer does not have to take that away from you.

Best wishes to you for better health and happiness through physical activity.

Lance Armstrong
Founder, Lance Armstrong Foundation
Five-time Tour de France champion

A WORD OF CAUTION

The Cancer Fitness program is based on scientific research. Detailed instructions and precautions are provided throughout the book, and it is important that you read each of them carefully. The recommendations given in this book are not meant to supplant or replace the advice of a health care provider who is familiar with your condition. We all have unique bodies, and it is critical for you to work in a partnership with your health care team. I advise you to check with your health care provider regarding precautions or contraindications to exercise that may be unique to you, your disease, or your treatment. The information and recommendations I provide are within the standards of practice at the time of publication.

CANCER
FITNESS

X MARKS THE SPOT:
A PERSONAL PERSPECTIVE ON CANCER AND EXERCISE

February 13, 1988. The x-ray marked the spot—non-Hodgkin's lymphoma. I heard the words and then couldn't take in the rest of what the doctor was telling me. As I gained a better understanding of what the diagnosis meant, I began to feel smaller and smaller as I pulled in with fright. My life was caving in, and I no longer felt like a free-spirited 24-year-old. I felt like the storm clouds had rushed in and were swirling around me and I was left blanketed in darkness. Alone, terrified, and confused, I was overwhelmed with decisions and emotion.

Like a horse with blinders on, I methodically plodded on through my final semester of nursing classes, the blinders blocking out what was happening to my life. Class met consistently at 8 A.M. and clinical assignment days began at 7 A.M. The regimen provided a distraction from the storm clouds, the only time the darkness from the clouds would lift to swirl above my head—though remaining an ominous presence that was always with me.

In a deliberate effort to minimize my fears and cope with the diagnosis, I called my cancer the "little problem." If it was a "little problem" it couldn't be too serious, right? The little problem changed my outlook on everything. I developed an intensity, concentration, and passion to pursue excellence or at least do my best and to do what I truly felt was important. What a change for a University of Florida partying Gator! Before my diagnosis I was your typical college kid, floating through life without many worries, doing my work, not exactly focused or driven.

I was always curiously interested in pushing the limits and exploring new frontiers, and when I graduated from nursing school I wanted a job that was cutting-edge and research focused. Somehow I didn't realize, or perhaps it was denial, that when I accepted a position in a bone marrow transplant unit that all the patients would have cancer. This was a difficult discovery and realization for me during my first week of work, because so many of the patients' concerns were all too close to my own personal struggle. To make matters worse, we were treating a woman my age with lymphoma who everyone thought looked like my twin. We not only looked alike, but we had the same sense of humor and similar likes and dislikes. I couldn't cope with taking care of her, much less seeing her or hearing her status in daily reports. I would go home after an evening shift feeling overwhelmed by the intensity and emotion of the day. Although I had always been a natural athlete and competed in tennis, swimming, and running in college, I was overwhelmed with everything in my life and got fat, depressed, and hopelessly out of shape.

I knew that I needed to do something; I needed to move! All my life, physical activity had always been freeing and centering for me. Bicycling had always appealed to me as the ideal form of sport—you got exercise, could go places fast—and a childhood dream had been to ride across the United States. So, at the urging of a friend, I started bicycling with the local group. Little did I know that Gainesville, Florida, was a winter training mecca for cyclists, and that I was riding with world-class cyclists. When I realized this, I was delighted, amazed, and incredibly motivated to pursue more time on the bike. I dived into bicycling with my newfound passion and enthusiasm and much to my surprise was achieving more than I ever imagined—my depression was resolving, I was losing weight, and I was winning races. I pursued cycling with zeal, enthusiasm, and intensity. I was determined to begin following the race circuit and to have a more flexible work schedule. My nurse manager was wonderful, and we negotiated a work schedule that allowed me to travel to races, set up a coaching and training business, and train to set three world records.

After many months of emotional struggle, I succeeded in sorting out my illness from those of my patients and learned that my experience gave me a different perspective and way of helping my patients. I credit cycling for helping me overcome this forbidding emotional challenge. My time on the bike often required a lot of concentration to stay with the group, but when I rode alone, I had hours to mull over the beauty and troubles of life. This time alone on the bike was like therapy. For me, exercise was therapy as I learned to sort out my cancer, my treatment, and who I was and what I wanted to do with the next year, three years, five years. And what if I had ten years? I learned from cycling the discipline and commitment that helped me not only get through cancer treatments but pursue my life passion of helping people to live beyond their cancer.

Over the next few years of work in the bone marrow transplant unit, I observed that some patients didn't seem to suffer as much as the others. The primary difference in these patients was that they got up and walked around their room or rode the stationary bicycle that typically sat in the corner of every room, most often being used as a clothes rack for raincoats or purses. The patients who followed their own exercise routine seemed physically and emotionally healthier. Often these patients were able to push their wheelchairs out of the hospital rather than being pushed out by someone else. As I observed the patients who were physically active, I realized that they seemed to be experiencing the same benefits that I had received from exercise. Exercise seemed to reduce their level of suffering, fatigue, weight gain, depression, and anxiety. Because I was so intrigued with this phenomenon, I decided to return to graduate school to pursue a degree that would give me the skills to become a researcher and conduct the studies necessary to investigate and, I hoped, confirm the link between exercise and cancer recovery.

I took a rather circuitous route to a doctoral degree in nursing, but along the way I learned that many health care providers were afraid to have cancer patients exercise and that little research had been done to study the effects of exercise on cancer patients. Building on my knowledge of exercise science (I earned a bachelor of science degree in this field at the University of Florida in 1985), it seemed logical that an exercise program could be developed that simply adapted exercise to fit the physical limitations of a patient with cancer. By now, I was an expert patient and oncology nurse, and I knew what needed to be done, but persuading a professor to support this research was no easy feat. So, I started trying to develop the knowledge that I needed, and along the way collected a number of academic degrees that, in hindsight, have been very helpful.

After some searching, I succeeded in finding a mentor who was supportive of my cancer and exercise research, and I began a wonderful new life combining my background in sports, and nursing and my fresh knowledge of research. The doctoral program allowed me to start formally testing my theory that exercise could reduce some of the side effects of cancer treatment. Ironically, my mentor, Lillian Nail, Ph.D., RN, FAAN, was a lymphoma and breast cancer survivor, but unlike me a certified couch potato. She brought a challenging perspective to developing this area of research and one that forced me to examine ways to make exercise during cancer treatment something that any patient could do. During my studies, I would take Lillian to the gym to exercise regularly. One of the many things she taught me was that some people need a hand, extra support, and guidance in learning to exercise and transitioning to become a regular exerciser. Coaching Lillian helped me develop insight into key elements that help people begin and stay with an exercise program.

My doctoral studies were interrupted in January 1995 by a recurrence. I was devastated and felt myself screaming inside, like the painting by Edvard Munch called *The Scream*, the familiar dreadful feeling of pulling in and shrinking as the dark storm clouds gathered. This time the clouds were darker and more ominous—the greenish tint of clouds before a violent storm or tornado. Dispair, disbelief.

I struggled to pursue my work during chemotherapy and

felt a huge obligation to exercise regularly since this was what I believed was the right thing to do and had helped me in the past. Besides, exercise was the tenet of my research. On the days following chemotherapy it felt impossibly hard to get up and move, but a walk or an attempt at a jog always made me feel better. I played tennis with IVs and PICC lines and felt stronger with every ball I hit, even if it went flying out of bounds. In 1997, I completed a Ph.D. in nursing at the University of Utah. Since that time I have been conducting research on cancer and exercise in newly diagnosed patients and in cancer survivors, always searching for ways to improve quality of life and reduce suffering.

Today, as I look back, I realize that I had no idea of the impact cancer would have on my life and my whole way of looking at the world. As distressing and horrible as the cancer experience was, I gained insight, strength, and the courage to pursue my dreams, which helped me to set three bicycling world records, win a national championship title, and become a leader in research on exercise for people with cancer. Although exercise is not customarily recommended or formally prescribed for cancer patients, I have learned through personal experience as a cancer patient, as an athlete, and now through careful scientific study with nonathletes that exercise can strengthen not only your body but also your soul.

My personal struggle with cancer, which includes recurrence and different courses of therapy, and my professional experience as an oncology nurse have given me a unique perspective to conduct research and teach others about managing their disease and healing. I hope the information in the following chapters will help you not only to begin an exercise program to strengthen your body and heal your soul but to realize your potential and live the fullest life possible.

There is strong scientific evidence that regular exercise is important during cancer treatment. Patients, young and old, thin and fat, fit and unfit who have participated in research studies provide consistent evidence that exercise is an important and all too often neglected part of the cancer treatment plan. Exercise can't make your cancer go away, but it certainly can help you look and feel better and have a better perspective and outlook on life.

CHAPTER I

CANCER AND EXERCISE: WHAT DOES THE SCIENCE SHOW?

There are many challenging side effects of cancer, but the most common and perhaps most frustrating is fatigue. Everyone has felt fatigue or tiredness during their lives, but the fatigue of cancer and its treatment is different. It is an overwhelming, all-consuming feeling that is not relieved with rest, and fatigue "attacks," sudden periods of utter exhaustion, come on unpredictably, making normal life activities an extreme challenge. Common sense tells us that resting more will make us feel better, but with cancer, rest often is not restorative. Although we may feel too tired to move, activity is key to avoiding the debilitating effects of inactivity, such as muscle atrophy (shrinking), reduced heart and lung function, and decreased endurance and strength to carry out usual activities. This chapter describes the physical and emotional effects of exercise on patients who are receiving cancer treatment.

EXERCISE IS SAFE

The science of exercise for cancer patients and survivors has evolved rapidly in the last decade. The first study of cancer patients and exercise was conducted in 1986, and it demonstrated that high-intensity aerobic exercise was safe for patients when they were receiving chemotherapy. These early researchers broke some of the barriers and fears that physicians and people in general had about cancer patients exercising during chemotherapy. Since that time, studies have repeatedly demonstrated that exercise is safe, well tolerated, and beneficial during chemotherapy, radiation therapy, immunotherapy, and bone marrow transplant. By building on decades of well-tested research studies in cardiac rehabilitation, the science of cancer and exercise research has progressed quickly, even though exercise prescriptions for cancer patients differ from recommendations for patients with heart disease.

FATIGUE

Cancer fatigue is a crushing, all-encompassing, incapacitating fatigue that is indescribable other than to say that it is completely draining.

—a 59-year-old man with stage IV prostate cancer

Fatigue is the number one side effect of cancer and its treatment. It is the most pervasive and disruptive side effect of cancer treatment and affects nearly 100 percent of patients. Researchers have observed that fatigue has a profoundly negative effect on quality of life. Although we don't know what causes fatigue, it is clear that exercise reduces fatigue. Research has shown that aerobic exercise during chemotherapy, immunotherapy, radiation therapy, and bone marrow transplant has a positive effect on reducing fatigue. In patients with metastatic disease, exercise has the same effect—it reduces fatigue.

The exciting news is that moderate exercise of short duration (as little as 10 minutes), performed at least every other day, is sufficient to reduce fatigue. For patients who are too tired, weak, or debilitated to exercise for a continuous amount of time, I have found that dividing exercise into short sessions of as little as 2 minutes is just as effective in reducing fatigue as struggling to complete one sustained period of exercise.

Figure 1 shows the differences in fatigue levels between patients with different types of cancer receiving chemotherapy who were assigned at random to exercise or to usual care activities. Moderate-intensity aerobic exercise has an immediate effect on reducing fatigue. Figure 2 shows the differences in fatigue levels between women with breast cancer who did and did not exercise while receiving radiation therapy for breast cancer. Although the fatigue level of the patients who exercised did not decline until the middle of treatment, by the end of radiation therapy the exercise patients had significantly less fatigue. I suspect that the delay before fatigue declines is because the exercise program in this study was of low intensity. Exercise is like a medication: the patients on the low-intensity exercise program may not have reached the therapeutic dose of exercise to reduce fatigue until the middle of radiation therapy.

Figure 1. Differences in fatigue between exercise and usual-care patients.

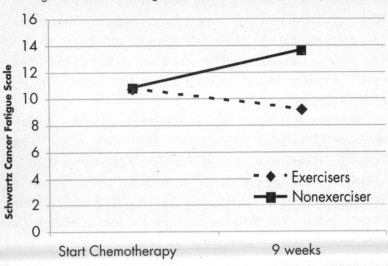

Figure 2. Differences in fatigue between exercise and usual-care patients receiving radiation therapy (RT).

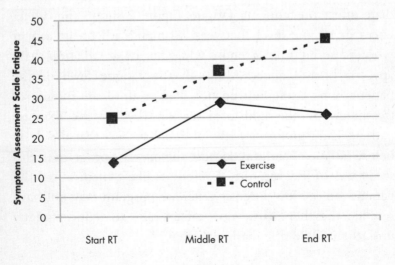

Mock et al. 1997

When we ask patients what their worst (or highest) level of fatigue is, those patients who exercise regularly report lower levels of fatigue, day after day, week after week. Patients who exercise also report lower levels of daily average fatigue, the fatigue that affects our ability to complete everyday activities. Those patients who exercise also tell us that the most important time to exercise is when they feel their worst. This counterintuitive information is hard to explain to someone who is too tired to move, work, or do other things that they value, but I have seen patients over and over go home and start to do basic exercises and return to see me a few weeks later, feeling not only a lot less fatigue but also a whole lot better about life.

AN EXERCISE CONVERT

Judith was a 60-year-old woman with stage II breast cancer. Her treatment included surgery, chemotherapy, and radiation therapy. She was not an exerciser before her cancer diagnosis. In fact, she was determined to avoid physical activity. She didn't like the way working out made her feel and couldn't imagine exercising after surgery and with all the unpleasant treatment that she was about to go through. I met her youngest son, Josh, in the clinic one afternoon. He expressed concern about his mother's cancer, her declining strength, and eventually said, "I want my mom to be at my wedding in June." We discussed the benefits of exercise. Josh expressed doubt his mother would change her sedate lifestyle, but much to his surprise she agreed to try an exercise program, if it didn't make her feel any worse. Judith started a gradual aerobic exercise program and after eight weeks told me, "After exercise I feel physically tired. It's a good tired, not the whole-body tired, consuming type of cancer fatigue." She continued to exercise throughout her treatment, and since she completed her cancer treatment, Judith has continued to exercise regularly. Exercise has become such an important part of her everyday life that she has organized a walking group and regularly invites women who are newly diagnosed with breast cancer to join her in her walks. Judith is an inspiration and role model for many patients looking to get though the challenges of treatment and feel their best.

REST—THE BIG MYTH

At the time of cancer diagnosis, most patients are not advised to start an exercise program. The usual dictum, given by well-meaning health care providers and friends, is to "rest" and "take care of yourself." For most people, this means sleeping more and being as inactive as possible to protect the body that yesterday may have felt quite well but today has deceived them. Research is showing us not only the benefits of exercise but also the deleterious effects of rest. The need to become inactive and rest is a myth!

Patients who earnestly follow the rest myth quickly become weak and debilitated. How much you are physically able to do varies by type of cancer treatment, but on average, patients who are inactive lose 5 percent of their functional ability during 7 weeks of radiation therapy, 16 percent during the first 9 weeks of chemotherapy, and 19 percent during high-dose chemotherapy for bone marrow transplant, usually in a 3- to 4-week time period. In my research, I have seen some patients lose as much as 35 percent of their physical ability. What this means is that as your physical ability decreases, simple activities such as walking up the stairs, grocery shopping, or walking to the car become more challenging and you feel tired more easily. Declines in physical ability have negative effects on emotional and social function and cause other serious physical problems, such as muscle wasting, bone loss, and declines in heart and lung function.

Being fit may not seem to be of great importance when you are confronted with the challenge of cancer and its treatment, but being physically fit is crucial to living a full life during and following treatment. Maintaining or increasing your physical fitness during cancer treatment can improve your quality of life, reduce the number and intensity of your side effects, and help in your overall recovery. Patients who are stronger are able to do more activities without getting so tired. If you become weak and debilitated during your treatment, it becomes much harder to continue with usual activities, such as dressing yourself, going to work or school, and socializing with family and friends.

Science is showing us that exercise has other positive physical benefits, too. Exercise is not a panacea for all the side effects you may experience, but it is a powerful intervention you can use to improve your physical and emotional health.

Luke was a 77-year-old man with recurrent lymphoma. When he was initially treated for his lymphoma, two years earlier, he received chemotherapy and radiation therapy and dutifully rested as the doctor told him to. Luke told me, "I rested so much I barely had the strength to get out of bed. I felt like a really old man as I tried to shuffle from place to place. I had to sit down every few feet to catch my breath and gather my energy. It took me over a year to get most of my strength back." Facing more therapy for his recurrent disease, Luke wanted to try a different approach. He enrolled in one of the exercise programs and learned the essential balance of rest and exercise. After Luke completed treatment he said, "In the darkness of cancer, I was amazed to be invited into an exercise program. I didn't have the terrible fatigue and weakness that I experienced during the first treatments. Actually, I was able to continue doing most of my activities like going to church, visiting with my family and playing poker with my old buddies. Exercise provided a ray of hope."

FUNCTIONAL ABILITY

I was worried about becoming too weak to work, but exercise kept me strong. Strong enough to push a cow around to examine it.

—a 42-year-old woman, a large-animal veterinarian,
with stage III malignant melanoma

Most health care professionals and patients do not expect their patients to become fitter and faster during cancer treatment. Exercise studies for patients receiving chemotherapy or radiation therapy consistently demonstrate that patients are able to get physically fit even with modest exercise. The 12-minute walk or run test is a measure of the distance an individual can cover in 12 minutes. The test is used to determine changes in functional ability and reflects heart and lung function. Patients with higher functional ability can cover more ground on the 12-minute walk/run, which means they are able to do more activities with less effort because they are more physically fit. Daily activities, like grocery shopping and keeping up the house, don't take all your energy if you are fit. If you improve your fitness you can do what has to be done and still have some energy to do the other activities that are important to you.

Figure 3 depicts the effects of a home-based moderate-intensity aerobic exercise program on functional ability in women newly diagnosed with breast cancer who are receiving chemotherapy. The sixty-eight women who exercised in this study were, on average, able to walk 15 percent farther on the 12-minute walk/run at the end of 9 weeks. In contrast, the usual-care patients, many of whom rested, were not able to cover as much distance and lost an average of 23 percent of their functional ability. Other studies of patients receiving

Figure 3. Changes in functional ability over 9 weeks.

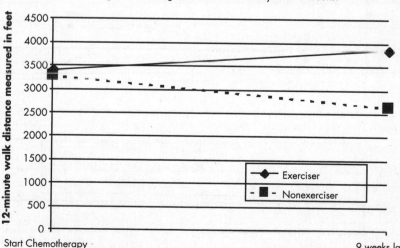

chemotherapy, radiation therapy, immunotherapy and bone marrow transplant have observed increases in functional ability ranging from 4 percent in a low-intensity walking program to 40 percent in a high-intensity interval-training program.

Figure 4 shows the results of a study that randomly assigned patients to aerobic exercise, resistance exercise, or usual care and followed participants for 6 months from the beginning of chemotherapy. The men and women in this study, who ranged in age from 20 to 78 years old, were all receiving a steroid and chemotherapy for treatment of a variety of different cancers. Although both exercise groups were more physically fit at 6 months, the patients in the aerobic exercise group had significantly greater gains in their functional ability, 16 percent on the average, compared to the resistance exercise group, who gained only 4 percent and the

Figure 4. Differences in functional ability between aerobic exercise, resistance exercise, and usual care.

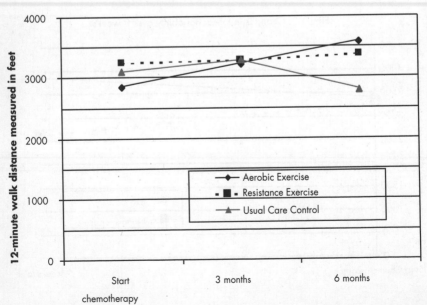

usual-care group, who showed average declines of 10 percent in their functional ability.

BODY WEIGHT

Weight gain is not what people expect when they start chemotherapy. Nonetheless, it is very common to see patients steadily gain weight during chemotherapy and for a time after treatment ends. Here again, exercise helps to prevent this frustrating side effect. Figure 5 shows the steady weight gain of women being treated for breast cancer who did not exercise compared to women who followed a moderate-intensity home based aerobic exercise program. Although the usual-care patients weighed more at the start of chemotherapy, they steadily gained weight over the four cycles of treatment. These women may have been less inclined to exercise because they were heavier. In contrast, the exercisers essentially maintained their body weight over time. I have observed this pattern of weight maintenance in both men and women who exercise, regardless of their type of cancer or type of treatment. Exercise as simple as walking to your mailbox or around the block may help to elevate your metabolism enough to keep the weight off.

> I thought the one benefit of chemotherapy is that it would help me get my figure back, but I gained over 9 pounds.
>
> —a 34-year-old woman with stage III breast cancer

Figure 5. Differences in body weight between exercise and usual-care patients.

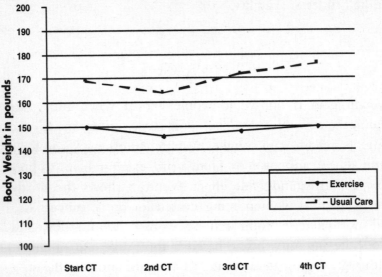

Weight gain may be frustrating and distressing in itself, and there is strong scientific evidence to suggest that the weight women with breast cancer gain during chemotherapy is difficult to lose and increases breast cancer survivors' risk of recurrent disease and development of a second breast cancer. Being obese or overweight increases any survivor's risk of other serious illnesses, such as diabetes, heart disease, high blood pressure, and bone and joint problems. Exercise not only can help to keep the weight off but is strongly associated with controlling blood sugar and reducing the risk of heart disease.

Weight loss is observed with some cancer treatments, such as interferon-alpha. Much to my surprise, my study patients who receive treatments that often cause weight loss and are assigned to exercise do not lose more weight than their nonexercising counterparts. Actually, patients who exercise while receiving interferon–alpha often report having a better appetite and less nausea. So, eating is not as much of a challenge for these patients.

BONE HEALTH

When faced with a life-threatening illness like cancer, we don't often worry too much about what might happen to us a few years down the road. We are worried about making it through the night or the next round of chemotherapy, and bargaining for a few more good months or years. Oncologists treat patients to cure them of their disease, often with little thought to the side effects that a patient may experience many years later. However, health care providers are becoming aware that some chemotherapy regimens used to cure various cancers, such as breast cancer and lymphoma, cause significant declines in bone density. These declines occur in men and women and in young and old patients but are most severe in younger women who were premenopausal when they started chemotherapy and are suddenly thrown into premature menopause by the chemotherapy. The cumulative effect of some medications, inactivity, and, for younger women, early menopause, is bone thinning, or osteopenia. In some patients the bone loss is so severe that the bones become porous, and the patient is classified as having osteoporosis. Both osteopenia and osteoporosis advance invisibly. Symptoms don't appear until bone loss is significant and the risk of fractures is high.

The good news is that exercise appears to reduce some of the bone loss that occurs during treatment. Studies show that patients receiving doxorubicin (Adriamycin), methotrexate and steroids, such as Decadron and prednisone, lose between 5 and 8 percent of lumbar spine bone density in the first year following treatment. In my current research, we are seeing average declines in bone density of nearly 8 percent in patients who rest and follow the usual-care advice of their health care team. In contrast, the patients who follow an aerobic exercise program have significantly less bone loss, only about 2 percent.

Exercise appears to play an important role in reducing the amount of bone loss during the first six months of chemotherapy.

Figure 6 shows the difference in bone loss between patients who followed aerobic and resistance exercise programs and those who followed usual care. Patients assigned to aerobic exercise lost significantly less bone mass (−1.8%) than either the resistance exercisers (−4.9%) or the usual-care patients (−6.2%). Although all exercise groups lost bone mass, when we looked at the differences by gender, the declines in bone density were greatest for pre-menopausal women but significant for men and post-menopausal women, too. Weight-bearing exercises, like walking and running, and exercises that stress and tug on the bones, like resistance exercise or weight lifting, stimulate bones to grow and balance some of the bone loss caused by treatment. Patients in the resistance exercise program did not show as much of a decline in bone loss as the aerobic exercise patients, possibly because the exercises were developed to increase muscle strength in general and may not have been sufficiently vigorous to stress the skeleton to preserve bone density.

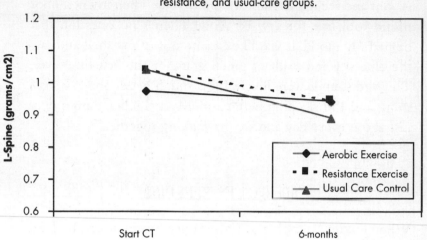

Figure 6. Changes in bone density between aerobic, resistance, and usual-care groups.

ANXIETY AND DEPRESSION

Anxiety and depression are common experiences during cancer treatment. Studies have demonstrated that exercise can reduce mild and moderate levels of depression and anxiety in the healthy population. Health care providers often prescribe moderate regular exercise for their patients with anxiety or depression. Similar effects of exercise are observed with cancer patients. Studies have observed that anxiety and depression increase during chemotherapy in patients who do not exercise but decrease in patients who exercise during treatment. Exercise can help patients feel more positive about life and in control of their health.

Sally was a divorced 50-year-old woman with stage II colon cancer. She had undergone surgery and was receiving a long course of chemotherapy that left her feeling drained, weak, and without interest in much life had to offer her. She told me, "I felt like life was closing in on me. I didn't want to go out and see my friends or do anything. Then my neighbor friend took me for a walk. Wow! There's no question that helped my mood. It was like I came out of my shell and saw the blue sky and brilliant green grass for the first time ever. The bird sounds were lovely. I feel much better about everything and I'm sleeping better too. My neighbor comes over just about every day and we go walking together."

DIFFICULTY SLEEPING

When anxiety is high and uncertainty looms, it can be hard to sleep. Sometimes the medications that are used to control nausea or are part of your treatment regimen can also cause insomnia. Whatever the cause, difficulty sleeping and insomnia are very common complaints during treatment that only make you feel more unsettled and on edge. Research with patients receiving a variety of different treatments has shown that exercise promotes better sleep. The reason may be that exercise reduces anxiety and depression so that it is easier to fall asleep, or simply that we need more activity to be able to rest efficiently. Either way, patients who exercise benefit by reporting less difficulty falling asleep and staying asleep.

SELF-ESTEEM

As shocking as it is to lose your hair, having to deal with people staring and saying inappropriate and sometimes outlandish comments makes the cancer treatment that much harder and can be a blow to one's self-esteem. Many factors contribute to how we feel about ourselves, and some of the changes from cancer treatment, such as alopecia (hair loss), a mastectomy, or other surgical change, may create increased feelings of vulnerability. The diagnosis of cancer may call into question all your goals and aspirations and make you wonder if they are reasonable or even feasible. Studies that examine the effects of regular exercise on the self-esteem of cancer patients report that exercise has a positive effect on improving self-esteem, building confidence and a positive attitude. Physical activity makes patients feel more focused, less "handicapped," and empowered. Clinically, patients who exercise tell me they feel stronger and better able to face the challenges and the uncertainties of cancer, and its treatment.

Jacob was a 19-year-old young man when he was diagnosed with stage II testicular cancer. Testicular cancer has a high cure rate, but nonetheless, any cancer at 19 years old is traumatic. Jacob's treatments and their side effects kept him from playing football with his friends and from his second semester of community college. He hated being back at home with his parents and felt depressed and frustrated by changes he could see in his body. Desperate to do something to get out of the house and exert his independence, he signed up for an exercise program. After spending at least two months lying on the couch watching television and playing video games, Jacob was determined to get stronger and followed the program regularly three or four days a week. Gradually he got stronger and could see his muscles redefine themselves. Jacob told me, "The exercise I did was in small steps but enough to strengthen my body and help me regain confidence in myself."

BODY IMAGE

Changes in body image are a disturbing consequence of cancer treatment, whether the change is related to weight changes, hair loss, or the disfiguring consequences of surgery. However, patients who exercise report lower levels of body dissatisfaction than their sedentary counterparts. This may be because physically active cancer patients report that exercise makes them feel "normal" and "healthy" and helps them to feel better about their bodies.

Many years ago when I was working as a registered nurse, I had a patient named Marla tell me that even though she was cured of her leukemia and very thankful for that, the scars on her body were a daily reminder of her illness and how it had changed her life. I realized at the time how deeply troubling the scars were for her but had no suggestions to help her. Recently I was reviewing the exercise program with Eric, a 30-year-old man with colon cancer. As he was exercising he told me, "Although you can't see the scar, I know it's there and that bothers me. It's a constant reminder. Exercise helps me to feel stronger, look better and feel attractive again." Eric's comment made me think of Marla, and I wish I had known then what we know now about the benefit of exercise for cancer patients.

OTHER BENEFICIAL EFFECTS

The presence and intensity of side effects negatively affect our quality of life. Studies have repeatedly demonstrated that exercise relieves nausea, improves appetite, reduces pain and diarrhea, and may even help cognition, or what many patients call "chemo-brain." Some people argue that patients who have fewer side effects are more likely to exercise and that the effects of exercise are not real, but this argument is weak in light of the numbers of patients who have been studied by different researchers around the world.

Patients who exercise while undergoing bone marrow transplant are discharged from the hospital sooner. We do not know why, but bone marrow transplant patients who exercise also appear to regenerate their white blood cells more quickly and require fewer red blood cell transfusions. This means these patients have fewer problems with infections and consequently are healthy enough to be discharged earlier from the hospital. Although no studies have examined the impact of fewer transfusions and infections and earlier hospital discharge on the cost of health care, it seems evident that exercise may have a cost-savings effect. The patients who exercise during and following bone marrow transplant also report less fatigue, more energy, and better fitness, which of course means that they are able to resume a normal life sooner than those patients who did not exercise and are suffering the consequences of prolonged inactivity—muscle weakness, declines in heart and lung function, and reduced energy and stamina. Unfortunately, it takes the body a long time and a lot of hard work to rebuild these losses.

Exercise is a timeless intervention that doesn't have to make you feel bad and can ward off some of the negative effects of the treatment and aging process while making you feel better right way. In this book you will learn how to develop an exercise program adapted to fit your own ability and physical limitations so you, too, can reap the benefits of exercise, get the most out of life, feel healthy, and improve your chances of long-term survival.

As you think about these scientific results, remember that research is dynamic. Currently, there are ongoing studies that will further refine these results and our understanding of the application of exercise in cancer treatment. We are living in an exciting time and should try to make the most of these remarkable findings to improve not only the quantity but also the quality of our lives.

KEY POINTS

- Maintaining or increasing your physical fitness during cancer treatment can improve your quality of life, reduce the number and intensity of your side effects, and help in your overall recovery.
- Exercise does not need to be hard or cause discomfort.
- Exercise done in short sessions, spaced out over the day, can decrease side effects from treatment.
- The functional ability losses from inactivity and rest take a long time to rebuild. These declines contribute to prolonged fatigue after treatment ends.
- Research is continuing to help us understand the effects of exercise during cancer treatment and survivorship.

CHAPTER 2

THE BASICS OF EXERCISE
DURING TREATMENT

The time before starting treatment is often the most difficult period, filled with dread and fears about the unknown. Once treatment starts, many patients feel better as they begin to know what to expect and how their body will react. Knowing how to deal with the side effects of treatment is a challenge and takes time but will certainly make you feel more in control. Everyone's reaction to treatment is different. Some patients may experience multiple side effects, others have very few, and we haven't perfected the crystal ball to be able to identify who will experience greater numbers or more severe intense side effects. These tips are designed to help you to feel better and to make it easier to start moving around and exercising.

WHEN AND HOW TO START

There's no time like the present to start moving. Pick a time of day that you feel your best and make the time to exercise. Dedicate and protect that time for your exercise. I've found that people are most successful with exercise if they do it early in the day, but there is no magical time. Find a time that works for you. You can plan for 5 minutes of exercise or 30 minutes of exercise, but be realistic about what you can do. The most common and defeating mistake is to think you can do more than you can and then push yourself too hard to accomplish your goal. Right now, you need to start far below your personal expectations. The goal is to feel good during and following the activity and not be uncomfortable. This is the way to make getting stronger fun and to see positive results.

If you have never been particularly physically active during your life, start off with walking, even if it is only around your hospital room for 3 minutes, and gradually increase your room walking or hallway walking to several times a day. As time goes on you will be able to walk 5 minutes 3 times a day and then 10 minutes all at once. I think you see how this builds. Don't make your heart pound or work so hard that your breathing sounds like a steam engine. Breathe through your nose and mouth, and feel yourself keeping an easy rhythmical pattern. As you get stronger and more accustomed to being active, you will be able to push yourself to go a little faster and for a longer amount of time, but when you're just starting and feeling pretty weak, start slowly. Give your body some time to catch up to the big ideas in your head.

Were you a regular devoted exerciser before your cancer

diagnosis? You too will need to cut way back on your exercise regimen. I recommend a 50 percent reduction in the length of time and intensity of your exercise. This may seem extreme, but your body is undergoing a huge challenge and the goal is to avoid overstressing the system. Start off easily and then gradually add time and intensity to your activity program after you see how your body reacts to treatment. I wouldn't expect that you will be exercising at your prediagnosis intensity level, but you certainly can play a game of tennis or participate in your favorite activity. Your goal should be to maintain as much of your fitness level as possible when you are receiving treatment. Don't let yourself become a couch potato.

EXERCISE AFTER SURGERY

Movement can usually begin soon after surgery, although it may be painful at first to move around much. Exercise after surgery needs to start slowly and gently, with a gradual increase in activity that is determined, to a large degree, by how your surgical wound is healing. The type and intensity of your exercise after surgery will also be determined and constrained by how your body is recovering from the surgery and anesthesia. Activity after surgery can be helpful in preventing some of the side effects of surgery, such as pneumonia and muscle wasting. Movement helps to keep your lungs moving air fully and reduce your risks for pneumonia while keeping your muscles strong.

If you had major abdominal surgery it may take a lot longer to start exercising than if you had a mastectomy or a sizable tumor removed for melanoma. The same principles apply, however: you must start slowly and listen to your body. If you have increased pain during or after the activity, slow down or stop. Immediately after surgery, it is important to work on stretching and limbering up the area again, but you need to get your doctor's approval before starting any kind of activity program. Most surgeons like to see their patients working on regaining their full range of motion, but depending on the type of surgery you had, it may take some time to heal before the surgical wound is ready for more vigorous exercise and lifting. Many surgical wounds take months to heal and attain their full strength. Even after a wound looks like it is completely healed, the skin's collagen (protein structures that support and hold the skin together) continue to build cross-links, which increase the strength of the skin at the site. Let your surgical team tell you when it is time to start exercising. The last thing you want to do in your efforts to improve your health are to make things worse by causing the wound to open or creating other problems, such as infection. If you feel your medical team is against exercise, ask them what they are concerned about, negotiate reasonable limits of exercise, and ask to work with a physical therapist who will guide you in slowly regaining your strength and flexibility.

EXERCISE DURING CHEMOTHERAPY, IMMUNOTHERAPY, AND RADIOTHERAPY

Chemotherapy, immunotherapy, and radiotherapy (radiation therapy) are treatments used to cure or control the cancer either by eradicating the cancer cells or by slowing down the growth or to keep a tumor in check and keep it from growing any further. Chemotherapy and immunotherapy drugs are not all the same. Some can be given by intravenous injection, and some can be given by mouth. Either way, the drugs enter the bloodstream and kill the cancer cells. Unfortunately, we have only half a handful of drugs that target only cancer cells. Most cancer chemotherapy and immunotherapy treatments have a broader effect, killing the cancer cells and also killing other rapidly dividing cells, such as those found in hair follicles and in the lining of the mouth and gut, which is why hair loss (alopecia) and mouth sores (stomatitis) are such common side effects.

All cancer treatments can cause unpleasant side effects. Before you can begin exercise you need to have your pain and nausea under control. This means that you need to learn to prevent the pain from getting bad or your nausea from getting out of control. How do you do this? Take your pain and nausea medication regularly, and review the tips in Chapter 3.

Early intervention and prevention of side effects will help you to feel better and allow you to begin making exercise part of your life and cancer treatment plan. If your medications are not controlling your side effects, tell your health care team and ask what other medications you could take. Don't wait until your next appointment, either! Call your nurse and explain what you are experiencing. Your doctor and nurse are your best source of reliable information. They should be able to provide clear advice for other nonpharmacologic remedies or a prescription to try a new drug or combination of drugs. There is no reason to "tough out" your side effects. If your side effect management plan isn't working, pursue another option. I find that many patients are often afraid to tell their health care providers that their nausea medication didn't work well or that they are continuing to have pain. Don't try to flatter your health care team by telling them everything is okay or to look like you can handle anything and everything. It's important to know that we have effective ways to manage side effects and that sometimes it takes several attempts to find the right drug or combination of drugs that work best for you.

Many of my patients find that exercise before chemotherapy, even their first course of chemotherapy, helps them to feel less anxious and more relaxed. Exercise not only reduces the anxiety and apprehension before treatment, it also gets your blood circulating, which makes it easier for the nurse to insert an intravenous catheter to draw blood or infuse chemotherapy. This of course makes the procedure much easier for you.

After my patients have been on chemotherapy for a few weeks, they often tell me that the most important time to exercise is when they feel their worst. Now, this may seem contradictory and may even sound crazy, but for many years, I have heard this over and over from patients. In general, I recommend that patients exercise at times of the day when they feel good, but sometimes when you are really pooped and your legs feel like lead, a little walk to the mailbox may be exactly what you need to wake up your body and feel better. Optimally, you will be able to exercise a little bit every day, or at least every other day. Regular exercise seems to be the key to reducing not only fatigue but also many other side effects patients experience during treatment.

EXERCISING DESPITE
TREATMENT-RELATED LIMITATIONS

Lymphedema

Lymphedema is a swelling of an arm or leg that results from extra lymphatic fluid collecting in the tissues. Most commonly we hear of women with breast cancer experiencing lymphedema or a swelling of the hand or arm after surgery to the axilla (armpit area). I have also seen other cancer patients with lymphedema in the legs, which makes walking and standing difficult and painful. For years, doctors have been telling their patients who have had surgery to the axilla for breast cancer or another disease to avoid picking up heavy items and not to carry a purse on the affected side. This conservative recommendation is given with the woman's best interest at heart, but slow, steady, systematic exercise can strengthen the arm and permit more normal use and function. In fact, no exercise study has reported that patients who exercise increase their risk for lymphedema. Dragon-boat paddling has become a popular fitness and fund-raising method for breast cancer survivors, and none of the clinical reports or research studies with these patients have reported increased incidence or severity of lymphedema. As a matter of fact, I believe that patients who exercise may have fewer problems with lymphedema, possibly because the exercise helps to keep the lymphatic fluid circulating, which may prevent some of the swelling. Studies that have focused on resistance exercises to strengthen the arms and shoulders have not observed higher rates or worsening of lymphedema, either. However, patients in these studies all started exercising slowly and gradually built up their endurance and strength. This is important to remember!

If you have had surgery to remove lymph nodes in the armpit or groin, or radiation therapy to that area, I recommend that before beginning your exercise program you measure your affected arm or leg. Write down the circumference of your arm or leg at the widest point and periodically remeasure it at the same point. This way you will be able to detect any size changes early, when lymphedema is easier to treat. Swelling or an infection can also cause lymphedema, so prompt evaluation and treatment are important. If the lymphedema is not caused by an infection, manual massage, lymphatic drainage, and compression garments can be used. Seeking the advice of a specially trained physical therapist can be most helpful in minimizing the long-term severity.

Peripheral Neuropathy

Peripheral neuropathy is a loss or change in sensation in an extremity. The changes usually start in the fingertips or toes and can affect the entire foot and hand. Many times the numbness gradually goes away over time after your treatments end, but sometimes there are long-lasting changes in sensation. Having numb hands or feet can be frustrating and can make walking and ordinary activity challenging. Some of my patients complain that they break more dishes because they can't feel the dish in their hands or that their balance and walking have changed. If you have numbness in your feet, does it change the way that you walk? Has it affected your balance? If your balance is changed, you may be safer choosing an activity in which you are less likely to fall. You may want to ride a stationary bicycle, swim, or walk with a friend or on a treadmill so that you can hold on if you lose your balance. Strengthening the core muscles in your hips, back, abdomen, and legs may help to reduce your chances of falling and prevent injury.

Infection

During chemotherapy and some immunotherapy treatments, your blood counts may become very low and put you at risk for infection. It is important to limit your exposure to heavily used public places, like gyms and spas, when your white blood cell count is at the nadir (low point). Simple measures like washing your hands regularly and trying not to rub your eyes or touch your face can help to reduce the chances of contracting some infections. If people are coughing, step back and give them space. Airborne viruses are easy to catch and difficult to avoid unless you are wearing a mask, and exercising with a mask on is hot and uncomfortable—certainly not something I would suggest. Masks are often recommended for patients to wear in public places following bone marrow transplant, but the use of masks is generally not necessary for patients receiving other forms of cancer treatment.

Skin Changes

Radiation therapy treatments can cause fatigue, skin irritation, itchiness, redness, peeling, and sometimes discoloration. Depending on where the radiation is focused, you may experience hair loss, vomiting, and diarrhea. Unless you are experiencing uncontrolled vomiting or diarrhea, these side effects should not limit your ability to exercise. If your skin is peeling and feels irritated in an area that could become sweaty, you may not want to exercise at an intensity level that causes perspiration, which may make your skin burn and feel more uncomfortable. Sometimes simply covering the area with a gauze pad can prevent problems resulting from perspiration.

Dizziness and Feeling Unstable

It is not uncommon for patients to feel dizzy and somewhat unstable on their feet. Most often this is related to poor hydration or nutrition. Unless you have been instructed to reduce or restrict your fluid intake, focus on staying well hydrated. Juice, soda, or whatever you prefer is fine; however, I think water is the best—no empty calories or sugar to rot your teeth. If you stay well hydrated you will feel better in everyday activities and during exercise. Being well hydrated is also better for your kidneys, which are filtering out a good bit of your chemotherapy.

When was the last time you ate? If you haven't eaten enough you may also feel dizzy and weak. If eating is a noxious task, try consuming high-calorie liquid beverages like Ensure or Boost with ice, thinned out with milk, or mixed in a blender and served as a milk shake. Adding protein powder to the mix is an almost invisible way to increase caloric intake easily. Drinking and eating are two of the simplest things you can do for yourself to feel stronger and healthier.

WHEN TO GO EASY
AND TAKE A DAY OFF

As you go through treatment, particularly chemotherapy, which is given in cycles generally ranging from 21 to 28 days, you will become aware of your energy, fatigue, and side effect patterns. Your exercise program should take into consideration when you may feel bad from treatment, which is usually the two to three days following chemotherapy. These days you may want to take off or do a very light activity.

Listening to your body and becoming aware of how you feel emotionally is important to your success in exercise. At times you may feel anxious, depressed, fearful, isolated, lonely, guilty, or sad. These are normal reactions to the tremendous life challenge of cancer. The stresses of diagnosis and treatment create fatigue. It is also important to try to distinguish whether you are feeling too tired to exercise because you are overwhelmed by the emotional strain or because you are truly tired. Exercise often helps to relieve emotional distress and stress in general. So, while you may feel too tired to move, it may be just the restorative activity your mind and body need.

We choose how we want to view and respond to the world. Try to adopt a positive outlook by thinking positively. This does not mean ignoring the scary realities in your life: it simply means looking for and acknowledging the positives in things. Thinking positively can have a powerful effect on your feelings of control over your situation, your feelings of helplessness, and your ability to appreciate the good things in life.

SETTING YOUR LIMITS

Just say no! Protect yourself from doing too much or doing things too soon. This may sound like a contradiction to my exercise advocacy, but evaluate your readiness to do activities like shopping or housework. Practice and be prepared to tell coworkers, family, and friends, "No, I can't do that right now." If you are a private person and don't want your colleagues to know about your cancer, you can still tell them no. Learning to say no is difficult, but it is an essential cancer survival skill.

If going to the grocery store will zap your energy, then ask friends to pick up a few things for you when they are at the store, or delegate the shopping to a family member. Make a list of chores that need to be done, and decide what you really have to get done. Then, think about who you can ask to do the chore(s). While on treatment, your job is to get well. If taking out the trash means you will be too tired to exercise later in the day, then ask someone to do that for you. Of course, eventually you will have to resume your usual activities; but you need to recover first and then you will be able to exercise and become fit and strong enough to complete your daily chores.

These limits, saying no, extend to your exercise program, too. If you are not feeling well, take the day off or exercise very lightly. If after two or three days of rest you still cannot exercise, you may need to step back and consider the possible reasons: (1) are you lapsing back into an inactive pattern, (2) do you have some other health issues that may indicate you should contact your health care team, or (3) have you forgotten your contract to make exercise a priority and to follow the Cancer Fitness program for 12 weeks?

EXERCISE PRECAUTIONS

Most physicians do not provide specific advice about exercise to their patients, but not for reasons related to your safety. Most physicians I know encourage their patients to exercise, they just don't tell them how or what to do. No exercise study with cancer patients and survivors to date has caused health problems for the participants. However, you need to be smart about your exercise habits. If you are starting a new pain medication that makes you sleepy, avoid participating in such activities as bicycling or those that require hand-eye coordination until you see how you respond to the medications.

There are no widely agreed upon or endorsed guidelines for exercise during or following cancer treatment. The following are some general guidelines for when to stop or skip exercise:

- Fever greater than 100°
- Early stages of an active infection
- Uncontrolled pain and/or nausea
- Dizziness or feeling unstable on your feet
- Shortness of breath in disproportion
  to the amount of work you are doing
- Chest pain or irregular heart rate
- Platelets less than 50,000 platelets per microliter
- Severe bone and joint pain

Early in the study of exercise and cancer, it was recommended that patients avoid exercise when their white blood cells, hematocrit, and platelets were at a slightly depressed level. These recommendations were meant to prevent patients from experiencing potentially deleterious effects from exercise, such as bleeding or infection, but we have learned that exercising with low blood counts is safe with proper caution and safety considerations. In the studies of patients receiving chemotherapy, either as outpatients or in the hospital during bone marrow transplant, all of the participants experienced low blood counts (white blood cells, platelets, and red blood cells) because they were receiving either chemotherapy or a combination of chemotherapy and radiation therapy. Both forms of treatment can reduce the number of blood cells circulating in our bodies and can cause anemia (low hemoglobin and hematocrit levels), increase the risk of infection when the white blood cells are low, and cause bleeding if the platelet count is very low. Remember, though, none of the studies showed more problems with bleeding or infection, and one study of patients undergoing bone marrow transplant actually found that patients who exercised required fewer blood transfusions, which means they experienced fewer problems with anemia. Curiously, the patients who exercised were also discharged from the hospital sooner. These findings are certainly intriguing, but the study was relatively small and the findings need to be replicated to confirm the effects of exercise on anemia and duration of hospital stay.

Even though we are learning that exercise is well tolerated during treatment, you need to use caution and some common sense if you are going to start an exercise program on your own. You need to be aware of your blood counts and perhaps keep a record of them. So, if your platelet count should fall below 50,000 platelets per microliter, you would know to consult with your physician about exercise and be very cautious in your exercise practices—avoiding exercises that have the potential for falls, or contact sports. Our platelets are necessary to stop bleeding; therefore, if you have an accident while exercising and your platelets are low, you put yourself at risk for a potentially serious bleed. This may not sound like a terribly dangerous problem, but if you fall off a bicycle or a horse and hit your head, the end result could be very serious. Try to stick with safer exercises such as stationary bicycling or rowing.

Problems related to anemia can be corrected with medications, such as erythropoietin (Procrit) or darbopoietin (Aranesp), or a transfusion. However, if you have a preexisting heart condition, lung problems, or are older (over 65 years), even mild anemia may aggravate other health conditions. Regardless of age, anemia makes it much harder to work and exercise because there are not enough red blood cells to carry all the oxygen your body needs to work. So, what may have been a light exercise workout last week may today seem like you are climbing Mt. Everest.

When you get your blood drawn for lab tests, be sure and request a copy of the results and of the normal values for the lab that does your blood work. By keeping a record of your blood counts, you can recognize when they are changing. Your health care team should be working with you to correct anemia and prevent prolonged periods of low white blood cells. At this time the only reliable way to correct very low platelet counts is by transfusion, but, fortunately most people don't require them often unless they are getting prolonged treatment or have other blood-related problems.

SARAH'S RETURN TO INDEPENDENCE

Sarah was a 46-year-old women with advanced breast cancer and diabetes. She got through chemotherapy but was severely limited in her activities from peripheral neuropathy in her feet and hands. She was unable to cook because she couldn't tell if a pot handle was hot, and she would drop dishes because she couldn't feel if they were slipping out of her hand. Walking was excruciatingly painful, and she leaned heavily on her walker as she slowly walked the 102 feet from her car to the office. When she arrived, Sarah was short of breath, her pain was worse, and she was exhausted from her tremendous effort.

Sarah was devastated by her physical condition and willing to try anything that could make her feel better. She began exercising in bed using TheraBands, which are like big rubber bands. Gradually she increased her strength. Since walking was so painful, she began a water exercise program. Over time, Sarah became much stronger and was no longer exhausted by walking from her car to the office. She worked with her doctors to find the right combination of medications for her pain, which also allowed her to exercise without feeling terrible. Talking to Sarah now is like talking to a new woman. She is more alert, energetic, and cheerful. Sarah proclaims, "I was in so much pain I wanted to die. I just couldn't stand doing anything. Water exercises and resistance exercises saved my life. Not just from a physical perspective, but emotionally too. Now I can be with my family and really be there, not just buried in my pain. I'm getting my life back."

MAGIC BULLETS

Regardless of the audience I address, a common question is "what should I eat to be fast or prevent fatigue or look better, or [insert your wildest wish]." The sad news is that there are no magic bullets except hard work, commitment, and dedication, which in time will lead to positive changes and achievement of your goals. Good nutrition is essential to being healthy, warding off many chronic illnesses, and achieving top athletic performance. Although we don't know what causes most cancers, we are beginning to see that there is a strong association between obesity, high-fat and low-fiber diets, smoking, and alcohol in the development of many cancers. This means eating a diet low in fat and including lots of fresh fruits and vegetables is important to maintaining and improving your health. A growing body of research has led organizations like the National Cancer Institute, the American Cancer Society, and other national task forces to develop recommendations and guidelines to prevent cancer, many of which include losing excess body weight, limiting fat intake to less than 30 percent of your total daily calories, consuming at least 5 servings of fresh fruits and vegetables, increasing your intake of high-fiber foods, and avoiding alcohol, smoked or salt-cured meats, and products containing nitrites.

At this time, nutritional scientists do not know enough about the potential benefits and risks of herbal products and supplements, such as Saint-John's-wort, shark cartilage, or vitamins, to make specific recommendations. For example, Saint-John's-wort is recommended to treat a variety of ailments, including insomnia, depression, wound healing, and burns, but we don't know much about this supplement and how it reacts to different types of chemotherapies. One of the problems is that we do not know the amount, or dose, needed for a beneficial effect. Another problem is that there is little regulation over the manufacturing of supplements, which means that you may be taking a product with no active ingredient or one that delivers far more than the amount listed on the label. However, the biggest concern with supplements is that the potential interactions with chemotherapy and immunotherapy are unknown, and the effect on the therapeutic outcome (your chances of survival) is also unknown.

In a recent study of lung and colon cancer patients, Saint-John's-wort was seen to increase the metabolism of irinotecan (Camptosar), a chemotherapy drug, and decrease the amount of the drug in the patient's body by about 40 percent. Even 3 weeks after the patients had stopped taking the Saint-John's-wort, their metabolism of irinotecan was impaired. The alterations in metabolism caused by Saint-John's-wort may have serious consequences on the effectiveness of treatment and survival. This is an example of one supplement that has actually been studied. Surprisingly, few supplements have been rigorously studied, which makes supplement use during cancer treatment somewhat risky at best.

Unfortunately, there are no quick or magical ways to lose weight nor perfect foods to prevent or cure cancer. Eating a healthy diet takes discipline and time to prepare. Many of my patients who change from eating a typical American diet that is high in fat and refined foods to a low-fat diet focusing on eating fresh, whole-grain foods tell me that if they exercise and make diet changes the exercise seems to help them continue to make healthy food choices. The combination of changing your exercise and eating habits seems to be complementary. Including family and friends in your lifestyle changes often makes adapting to your new routine easier.

I've never been an athletic person and have always looked for the easy way to lose weight, the magic pill. Now, I understand how important fitness is to every aspect of my life.

—Toni, 56 years old, with colon cancer

ANSWERS TO SOME COMMON QUESTIONS

The following are common questions people ask about aerobic and resistance exercises.

What shall I wear?

Ah, the fashion question that we all worry about and use as a way to hide the real question: how will I look? Regardless of your activity, unless of course you are swimming, wear loose comfortable clothing and a comfortable well-cushioned pair of shoes. The new synthetic fabrics are breathable and cool. If you are going walking, plan to dress in layers so you can regulate your body temperature. If the weather is warm, bring a bottle of water.

Is it better for me to follow aerobic or resistance exercise?

From a cancer treatment and symptom management position, I'm not sure that we have enough information to say that one type of exercise is better than another. I think the answer lies in how you are physically and emotionally. If you are confined to bed, then starting a resistance program will smooth the progress of your long-term recovery and get you back on your feet sooner. If you have been curled up on the corner of the couch "taking care of yourself," you may benefit most from aerobic exercise. Aerobic exercise will help you to get your endurance back so that you have enough strength and energy to get through the day. If you have time and can make the commitment, a combined aerobic and resistance program may give you the most satisfying results. The resistance exercises will quickly reshape and strengthen your body, the aerobic exercises give you the endurance that is essential to getting your full life back.

I've tried to exercise before but I get achy and sore and discouraged.

It sounds as though you are pushing yourself too hard. If you go from resting on the couch or simply doing your everyday activates to working out several days a week, you will be sore. I don't want you to start exercising that vigorously. Start slowly. Set reasonable and attainable goals, and have a plan. Write down your exercises in a log so that you can see why you might be getting sore and achy—perhaps you've increased your exercise time or intensity or are doing more resistance exercises. If you start a sensible, gradually progressive exercise program, I expect you will succeed.

If I do resistance exercises like lifting weights, will I get big muscles?

This is a common and needless worry, particularly for many women beginning a resistance exercise program. Women do not have the high levels of testosterone necessary to build large muscles, and women have less muscle mass than men. The fact is that as you get stronger your body will change. Fat takes up far more space, almost as much as five times more space, than muscle. So, when you steadily and consistently do resistance exercises, or lift weights, you will build stronger muscles as you replace the fat. In the end, however, you will look leaner. The ironic thing is that as you become stronger your weight may not change because muscle weighs more than fat, but your clothing will fit you better.

Can I change my body shape just by walking or doing other aerobic exercise?

If you consistently follow an aerobic exercise program for a long time, you will see changes in your muscles and physique, but not as quickly as you would if you were following a resistance exercise program. Aerobic exercise may help you to lose weight, but you will need to devote a considerable amount of time to exercise and diet modification. If you want to transform the shape of your body, start the Cancer Fitness resistance exercise program.

Is one form of exercise better for older people?

We all lose strength if we don't use our muscles, and as we age we lose our muscle mass. The loss of muscle mass and strength often leads to weakness, which contributes to feelings of fatigue and puts us at greater risk for falls and physical disability. Older people benefit from resistance training and aerobic exercise just as much as younger folks. Regardless of your age, you need to start an exercise program slowly and pace yourself so that you don't get hurt. Many exercise studies with older adults, over 70 years old, have shown us that exercise is safe and that older people become stronger and fitter with physical activity. There is little doubt in my mind that exercise is probably the best way to retain youthfulness and vigor.

Is aerobic or resistance exercise better for helping my mood?

From my clinical experience, both resistance and aerobic exercise make people feel better, and research studies suggest the same. Any form of physical exercise can reduce anxiety and improve your mood and outlook on life.

How do I exercise if I have a physical disability or limitation?

In different sections of the book I have described how to exercise if you are confined to bed or a wheelchair or have limitations because of peripheral neuropathy or lymphedema. What I hope you learn from this book is to focus on your ability and to learn that with a little flexibility, creativity, and determination, you can work around, and with, varying disabilities to find new and sometimes different ways to reach your fitness goals. Don't let your limitations become an excuse and a barrier to your quest for better health during and following cancer.

CONCLUSIONS

Science has made tremendous strides in the development of drugs to control the side effects of cancer treatment, such as nausea and pain. Take advantage of these medications; not only they will help you to tolerate the optimal treatment, but they can speed your recovery following treatment by allowing you to be more active. Logic, common sense, and the patience to start slowly will make it possible for you to follow an exercise program to improve your physical and emotional health. Exercise is safe for you when you are receiving cancer treatment if you listen to your body and pay attention to your blood counts.

> Exercise opened my eyes to the possibilities in my life, not just by regaining my body, but by giving me hope and the strength and courage to see I could get through this and make other positive changes in my life.
>
> —Jose, 48 years old, with lymphoma

CHAPTER 3

MANAGING YOUR SIDE EFFECTS

One of the biggest challenges of cancer treatment is learning to manage the numerous unpleasant side effects, and before you can even think about starting an exercise program during treatment you need to learn these skills. Although exercise during treatment has significant benefits, you won't be able to enjoy those benefits if pain and nausea are preventing you from exercising. Over the course of treatment we eventually learn ways to manage our side effects, but the sooner you learn effective strategies the better you will feel. Exercise can reduce nausea, fatigue, and other side effects, but it is important to learn a variety of ways to manage these and many of the other unpleasant sensations you may experience.

If you learn to manage your side effects aggressively and the optimal times to use these strategies, you will not only feel better but also be able to enjoy the benefits of exercise. The previous chapters explained how participants in research studies who exercised were physically healthier, calmer, and happier and enjoyed better concentration than those who did not exercise. This chapter will provide you with clear practical advice about how to manage your side effects from treatment and specific questions you may want to ask your doctor.

LEARN TO MANAGE YOUR SYMPTOMS

Zachary was a 29-year-old body builder with stage III testicular cancer. We met a few hours before he received his first dose of chemotherapy, a rigorous regimen that would entail many hours every week of intravenous chemotherapy infusions. He was a national champion wrestler and had aspirations to make the U.S. Olympic team. The first course of treatment caused severe nausea and vomiting that lasted for many days. He lost over 9 pounds in 2 weeks and became weak and incredibly fatigued. I saw Zachary during his third week of treatment; he was scared and frustrated, feeling down and truly dreading the next treatments. Zachary told me, "I didn't want to call the doctor because he told me I would have some nausea, but I just couldn't imagine it would be this awful. I can barely walk across the room."

I reviewed his medications with him and when to take them. As it turns out, Zachary was waiting until he felt nauseated to take the pills, which also meant that he was too nauseated to drink or eat much—afraid of the consequences. I instructed him to start taking the antiemetic (medication to prevent nausea and vomiting) on a regular schedule, not to wait until he felt nauseated, and to drink and eat small meals regularly. At the end of a week he telephoned me to report on how he was doing. He said, "I still have mild nausea, but I don't have the weakness and I can eat and drink if I take in a little at a time. I feel best if I eat and drink something every hour or two. Best of all, I'm now doing some stretching and very light, easy weight lifting." Over the next few weeks, Zachary learned to recognize the early signs of nausea and dehydration and learned when to start taking his antiemetics. He regained most of the weight that he had lost and was able to regularly do his "easy" workouts of weight lifting, stretching, and light jogging.

MANAGING THE COMMON SIDE EFFECTS OF TREATMENT

Fatigue

Fatigue is the most commonly reported side effect of cancer treatment. It is associated with every type of treatment and type of cancer. Fatigue is an overpowering lack of energy that can affect every part of your life. Cancer-related fatigue is not the same kind of fatigue as the fatigue you felt before cancer. It is a more extreme feeling of exhaustion. You may feel weak, have difficulty concentrating, and encounter problems getting your usual activities done. To make the experience of fatigue even more frustrating, it is not relieved with rest: common sense tells us that if we take a nap or sleep a little longer we will feel better, but this is not the case with cancer-related fatigue. Surgery, chemotherapy, radiation therapy, lack of sleep, poor appetite, inactivity, stress, and worry can all contribute to fatigue.

Fatigue is an important side effect that you should report to your health care team. Feelings of fatigue do not mean that your cancer is getting worse or that you are not responding to treatment. Fatigue is a common side effect of treatment, and there are ways to help you manage your fatigue. You should plan to tell your health care provider how your fatigue affects your daily routine activities and your ability to think and concentrate.

Try to determine your pattern of fatigue. Are there times of the day that you feel better or worse? If you are receiving chemotherapy, you might consider planning activities in the days before your next treatment, when you should be feeling better. Plan to do quiet activities at home two or three days after chemotherapy.

Commonsense Tips to Manage Your Fatigue

- When do you feel your best? Try to plan activities around your peak energy times. For example, if you feel best in the morning, plan your activities around that time.
- When you feel your best, pace yourself. Doing too much often causes a series of days of profound fatigue before you feel good again. This yo-yo pattern of fatigue is frustrating. Make plans, and pace yourself.
- When is your energy at its lowest? Plan time for a rest or quiet time, before you become too exhausted. Fifteen to twenty minutes of quiet time can help you regain some energy and feel more centered.
- Make a list of chores that need to be done. Prioritize. Decide which tasks are the most important

and which you may want to do yourself. Do those chores first, and then delegate the other tasks to someone else.

- Learn to ask for help, and accept it. People are more than willing to help! Be clear and tell them what they can do to help you. Give them specific chores, such as taking out the trash, doing yard work, picking up groceries, sweeping the porch, or driving you to doctor's appointments.

- Try not to be a couch potato. We know that inactivity leads to muscle loss and that muscle loss can lead to fatigue. It's a vicious cycle that you can stop to some degree simply by increasing your physical activity.

- Exercise, such as walking a short distance, can be helpful to increase energy, improve mood, and decrease fatigue. Follow the instructions in the next chapters.

- Good nutrition is important. Your body needs fuel from food to make energy. Small, frequent, nutritious meals are easier on your body than large meals or junk food.

- If you drink caffeine or alcohol, drink in moderation. These drinks can be dehydrating.

- Drink at least 8 to 10 glasses of fluids, including water, each day.

- Try to reduce stress in your life.

- Engage in relaxing activities, such as listening to music, reading, visual imagery, light massage, or exercise.

- Relax before going to bed at night by reading a book or taking a bath.

- Try to follow a regular sleep routine. A consistent nightly regimen can help your sleep.
- If you are not sleeping well, speak with your health care team. As all know, lack of sleep will cause more fatigue.

Treatments for Fatigue

Although we do not know all of the causes of fatigue, we do know that anemia (a lack of red blood cells often caused by cancer treatments or the cancer itself) is a common and correctable cause of fatigue. Blood transfusions or the use of medications that stimulate red blood cells to grow (erythropoietin [Procrit] or darbopoietin [Aranesp]) are safe and effective ways to correct anemia and help to reduce fatigue. Other causes of fatigue are not as clear but are observed clinically. Studies are under way to examine the effects of stimulants and antidepressants on reducing the cognitive effects of fatigue, also called "chemo-brain," that are so annoying and keep us from remembering words, phrases, and what we were going to say. Chemo-brain is not only a problem during treatment but can affect some people for months and even years after treatments have ended. There is still a lot we have to learn about fatigue and how to prevent and manage it. Perhaps in the not too distant future, fatigue will be an old problem that is an annoying but controllable, or perhaps even preventable, side effect of treatment.

Why Take Fatigue Medications?

"More medications? Why? Can't I just deal with the fatigue?" These are common questions I hear from people beginning treatment who are feeling overwhelmed by the entire experience and the number of medications they must take. There are many important reasons to treat fatigue. They include (1) if you improve your tolerance for treatment, it may mean that you are able to take the full dose of treatment and have a better outcome; (2) early research suggests that by correcting the fatigue associated with anemia may make some treatments more effective, which means you may have a greater chance for a cure or remission, and (3) there is clear scientific evidence that by reducing fatigue you will be able to enjoy a higher quality of life, which may be the most important reason of all.

PAIN

No one wants to have pain, but people have misconceptions about what pain means and how to treat it. Pain has been studied for many years, and we know a lot about how to manage it safely and effectively. Here are some basic facts about pain that are critical for you to know and understand.

- Pain does not mean your cancer is getting worse or that your treatment is not working.
- Pain medications work best when taken on a regular basis, what we call "around the clock."
- Pain is easier to manage when it is mild. When pain is severe, it is more difficult to control and

often requires more pain medication to get it under control.

- Addiction rarely occurs when patients have pain. Pain is a real reason to take your medication. Most drug addicts are self-medicating and do not have a medical reason to take pain medication. Drug addicts are taking the medication to get "high," not to control pain.

- Your body can develop a tolerance to the pain medication. When your pain medication is taken consistently for a period of time, it may not be as effective as it was when you first started taking the drug. Drug tolerance is easily managed by increasing the drug dose, using a different medication, or even adding a new medication. Often, two medications together work better than one medication alone.

- Tolerance to your pain medication is not addiction! It is your body's natural response to the pain medication. When your pain begins to subside your use of pain medication will too.

Why Do I Have Pain?

There are many reasons you may experience pain. Pain can come from the cancer tumor(s) pressing on bones, nerves, or organs. Treatment can also cause pain, for example, (1) radiation therapy can cause skin breakdown and reddening, called radiation dermatitis; and (2) chemotherapy can cause mucositis, reddening, and ulcers and sometimes even an infection in your mouth and throat. You may also experience everyday pain from headaches, arthritis, and muscle strains.

What Can Happen If I Do Not Take Pain Medication?

If you have pain you may not want to move much or be as active. Being active is very important in the recovery process. There are many risks associated with being inactive and staying in bed. These risks include muscle weakness, increased risk of infection, reduced heart and lung efficiency, poor sleep, depression, anxiety, and increased fatigue. If you have untreated pain or pain that is poorly controlled, you may feel anxious, irritable, and even depressed. Controlling your pain can help to keep you active and improve the quality of your life.

Communicating with Your Health Care Team

A key to your pain management is being honest and straightforward with your health care team about your pain. Use the tips included in this chapter. Do not minimize how you are feeling.

Types of Pain Medication

There are many different drugs to manage pain. *Nonopioids* include acetaminophen (Tylenol) and nonsteroidal anti-inflammatory drugs, such as naprosyn (Aleve) or ibuprofen (Motrin). These medications are prescribed for mild to moderate pain. Nonsteroidal anti-inflammatory medications are often prescribed for pain associated with swelling, bone metastasis, and muscle strains. *Opioids* are drugs that include morphine, hydromorphone, oxycodone, and codeine. These medications are used for moderate to severe pain and are sometimes used in combination with nonopioids. *Antidepressants* and *anticonvulsants,* such as amytriptyline, imipramine, neurontin, and phenytoin, are commonly used for the tingling or burning pain associated with nerve pain. *Steroids,* such as Decadron and prednisone, can be prescribed for a variety of reasons. Steroids can reduce bone pain or pain caused by swelling and inflammation.

Ways to Take Pain Medications

Pain medications, just like most other medications, can be prescribed by mouth (orally), by vein (intravenously, IV), by rectum in a suppository form, or by a patch on the skin (topically). How you take your pain medicine depends on your needs and the type of medicine prescribed. It is important to take the medication regularly and not to wait until you have pain. Ideally, you want to prevent the pain. Remember, you will not become addicted to your pain medication. You will gradually reduce your usage as your pain goes away.

Common Side Effects of Pain Medication

It is most important to understand that side effects tend to subside over time. Some common side effects of pain medications include constipation, nausea, and sleepiness.

Constipation can occur when both nonsteroidal anti-inflammatory drugs and opioids are taken. Prevention is the best approach. You can reduce constipation by increasing your fluids (juice and water) and eating a diet high in fruits and vegetables. A stool softener or fiber supplement at bedtime may also be helpful. Laxatives can also be added to your regimen. Being active and including exercise in your daily routine is important to keep your bowels moving.

Some pain medications can cause nausea, a queasy stomach, and sometimes even vomiting. Although this side effect generally subsides after one or two days, you may want to take a medication to stop the nausea. Let your health care team know if this happens to you. Sometimes changing your dose or the medication can help.

Sleepiness or drowsiness is a side effect of some pain medication. This side effect usually goes away after a couple of days. Talk to your nurse or doctor if the sleepiness persists and is bothersome. If this continues you may need an adjustment in your medication dose. If you are beginning a new medication you might want to try to start it at the end of the workweek so you will feel better on Monday and any potential side effects will not affect your work.

Certain medications can slow your breathing rate. Concerns about this side effect should be discussed with your nurse or doctor.

Nonmedication Approaches to Pain

There are many nonpharmacologic ways to reduce and control your pain. Some of these techniques are simple and can easily be learned. Breathing exercises, relaxation, imagery distraction, and massage can be helpful skills to reduce or control your pain.

Sometimes when we have pain we change the way we breathe. It is important to take slow, deep breaths in and control your breath as you breathe out. Holding your breath or breathing very fast can make your pain worse and make you feel nervous and lightheaded.

Learning relaxation and imagery techniques can be helpful not only in learning to cope with your pain but also as a strategy to manage your stress.

Reading a book, talking to friends, or watching TV or a funny movie are good ways to get your mind off how you feel and distract yourself from your discomfort.

Applying hot or cold packs to the area that is painful can decrease muscle spasms and other painful sensations. Cold tends to numb an area of pain, which can be a very effective way to manage pain. Heat can help to reduce muscle spasms.

Massage can be used to the area that is painful to help relax painful and tight muscles. Massage can be learned or be done by a massage therapist. Getting enough rest is important. When you are well rested it is easier to tolerate pain. Feeling rested helps you to have a more positive and open view of life.

Other Approaches to Pain Management

All of the following pain management approaches require supervision and prescription by licensed practitioners. These methods can effectively reduce and control pain. *Acupuncture* can be effective in reducing pain, if properly done. *Biofeedback* is a technique that you may be able to learn to help you control your pain. *Transcutaneous electrical nerve stimulation* (TENS) uses small electrical currents to interrupt pain sensations.

Radiation therapy can be prescribed to control certain types of cancer pain, especially from bone metastasis. Radiation therapy helps to reduce and control pain by shrinking the size of the tumor. *Nerve blocks* and *neurosurgery* can be helpful to block or cut the pain or actually remove the source of the pain, such as when a tumor is pressing against a nerve.

Learn to Describe Your Pain

It is important to learn how to describe your pain clearly. The way you describe your pain helps your health care team determine the best way to treat it. The following are some important characteristics of pain that can be helpful to describe how you feel.

- Where is the *location* of your pain?
- How does your pain *feel?*

Dull	Sharp
Throbbing	Burning
Stabbing	Tingling
Radiating	Crushing
Sudden	Intermittent
Constant	Shooting

- What time is your pain at its worst?
- Does the pain wake you up?
- Do certain activities make it worse or better?

Walking	Sitting	Coughing
Lying down	Lifting	

- What medication are you taking? How much? How often?
- Learn to rate the *intensity* of your pain on a scale of 0 to 10 (0 = no pain and 10 = worst possible pain). This will help both you and your health care team determine how well your pain is being managed and if changes should be made. The following is an example of a pain scale.
- *My level of pain* today *is:*

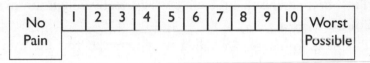

No Pain	1	2	3	4	5	6	7	8	9	10	Worst Possible

Although there are many different types of pain, the sensation of pain, if untreated, can make you feel exhausted, anxious, and unable to think clearly or move comfortably and can wreak havoc on your quality of life. There are many safe and effective ways to treat pain. Regularly taking pain medication will not lead to addiction; in fact the medication may help you to lead a more active and full life. Learning to describe where you have pain, when it occurs, how it feels, and how bad it is helps you to work with your health care team to manage your pain and improve the quality of your life.

NAUSEA

Nausea and vomiting are common side effects of many cancer treatments. Both chemotherapy and radiation can cause nausea. Sometimes the combination of chemotherapy and radiation therapy can cause more nausea then if you were given chemotherapy or radiation therapy alone. Nausea with chemotherapy can begin the day of treatment and sometimes lasts for several days. The nausea associated with radiation is different. You probably will not experience radiation-related nausea unless you are receiving radiation to your abdominal area. If you are receiving radiation to the abdomen, chest, or spine, you may feel nauseated or vomit a few hours after your treatment. Some people find that the nausea takes a few days to develop and gradually builds over the course of treatment. The good news is that there are very effective medications to control nausea.

Drugs for nausea are called antiemetics. If you are receiving chemotherapy or radiation therapy that causes nausea and vomiting, you will be given a prescription before you leave the clinic. It is important to take the antiemetics prescribed to control any nausea you may experience at home. If you continue to have nausea and vomiting and you are taking the medicine as prescribed, you should call your health care team.

How to Control Nausea

Prevention is the best way to control nausea. Take the antinausea medication (antiemetic) as prescribed. Some of these drugs are expensive. If your health insurance does not cover these medications, tell your health care team. Many times a different drug may be prescribed or your health care team can work out cost issues with the pharmacy or the pharmaceutical company that makes the drug.

If you are unable to take the antinausea medication by mouth because of vomiting, notify your health care team.

Antiemetics can be given in other ways—by vein or by rectum in suppository form. If you feel your nausea could be better controlled, tell your health care team. Usually your dosage can be increased or the medication can be switched or combined with another drug.

Tips to Reduce Nausea

- Try eating foods and drinking beverages that you have tolerated at other times when you were nauseated. People usually find that bland foods, such as dry crackers, ginger ale, and rice, are easy to take.
- Eat cold or room temperature foods. Avoid hot foods, which can have stronger odors that often make nausea worse.
- Avoid fatty, fried, spicy, or very sweet foods. These types of foods may increase your nausea.
- Do not eat your favorite foods when you have nausea. You may develop a dislike for those particular foods.
- When at all possible, have someone else do the cooking when you are nauseated. Stay away from the kitchen and cooking odors.
- If you routinely have nausea after chemotherapy, prepared frozen meals might be helpful.
- Drink an adequate amount of fluids. Often chemotherapy makes our sense of taste change, so find a beverage that you like. This may be water, a carbonated drink, juice, or an electrolyte drink such as Gatorade.
- Keep your mouth clean. Brush your teeth at least

twice a day. Rinsing your mouth with salt water can help remove unpleasant tastes.

- Some people find that relaxation techniques help reduce nausea.
- Acupuncture is helpful for some people who experience severe nausea.
- Acupressure wrist bands can also help some people with nausea.

When to Call Your Health Care Team

- The nausea stops you from doing your daily activities.
- You cannot keep anything down.
- You are vomiting and you lose more than two pounds in one day. You may feel thirsty, and your mouth might be dry because you have lost a lot of water.
- You are vomiting and your urine is dark yellow, or you are not going to the bathroom as much as you normally do.
- You feel lightheaded, dizzy, or confused.
- What you're throwing up is dark or looks like coffee grounds.

MUCOSITIS OR MOUTH SORES

Cancer and cancer treatments can cause mucositis, or mouth sores, and thrush, white patches caused by a yeast infection. Both chemotherapy and radiation therapy work by targeting and killing the rapidly growing and dividing cells, such as the cells that line your mouth. Cancer therapy can leave your mouth red and painful. Your mouth plays an important role in your health.

Examine your mouth at least once a day. Use a flashlight to look at your mouth and tongue in the mirror. Look for any sores or red or white patches.

How To Prevent Problems with Your Mouth

- Clean your teeth, gums, tongue, and roof of your mouth, even if it is sore. Use a soft brush or sponge-type swab that is very soft.
- Rinse with a saltwater or baking soda solution (½ teaspoon of salt in 8 ounces of water) every 1 to 2 hours. Often a cold solution will make your mouth feel better, too.
- Hold the toothbrush or swab with the grooves at an angle to your gum line. This helps you to clean well between your teeth.
- Gently brush your gums, tongue, and top of your mouth.
- If you wear dentures and they feel uncomfortable, you may want to take them out at night. If you are experiencing mouth sores, try to wear your dentures only while eating.
- Keep your lips coated with a water-based lip moisturizer.
- If your mouth is dry, drink water and other fluids, such as nonacidic juice or electrolyte drinks (e.g., Gatorade) frequently throughout the day. Sugarless

hard candy or gum can help keep your mouth less dry. Artificial saliva is also available and can be used frequently.

What to Avoid

- Chewing tobacco or smoking cigarettes, cigars, or a pipe.
- Drinking alcoholic beverages (beer, wine, or hard liquor).
- Strong mouthwashes or products with hydrogen peroxide that may actually burn your mouth.
- Do not floss your teeth if your platelet count or white blood cell count is too low (less than 50,000 platelets per microliter or as directed by your doctor) or if it causes pain or bleeding.

What to Do

If your mouth is too sore to eat comfortably, ask your health care team for advice. You may be given a medication to numb your mouth before eating meals and washing your mouth. These medications, such as Xylocaine, can be applied to the areas that hurt, swished around in your mouth, and spit out. Cool foods, such as ice cream and cool drinks, are usually easier to eat. Be careful with foods that are hot and spicy.

Take pain medicine at least 60 minutes before meals. If your mouth hurts all the time, you may benefit from a more aggressive pain relief plan or a medication that is taken around the clock. Talk with your health care team about ways to manage your pain. If you feel you need a stronger medication, consult with your health care team.

Infections can make mouth pain worse. If you have white patches or very red areas, you should check with your health care team for further instructions to help with your mouth sores. If bleeding occurs, put gentle pressure with ice on the area.

Eating with a Sore Mouth

Try to eat a well-balanced diet. Good nutrition is important in the healing process. This may sound simple, but when your mouth hurts, eating is an unpleasant challenge. Eating small frequent meals is often easier than eating three big meals. Drink at least 2 and ½ quarts of water per day (about 8 to 10 glasses), unless you have been told specifically to limit fluids. Try to avoid food that is hot, rough, or coarse, highly spiced or acidic, or any other foods you find irritating. Cold foods like Popsicles, milk shakes, or cold soups may be less painful to eat and easier to take.

Reasons to Call Your Health Care Provider

- Temperature greater than 100.5°F
- Bleeding that does not stop with gentle pressure
- Signs of infection in your mouth, such as white patches, redness, blisters, or ulcers
- Increasing soreness or pain
- Difficulty swallowing

CONSTIPATION

Constipation can occur from lack of activity, change in diet, or decreased fluid intake. Some medications can also cause constipation. Being constipated can cause significant belly pain and discomfort. The following are some tips to help you keep your routine bowel schedule.

- Drink plenty of fluids, at least 8 to 10 glasses per day.
- Eat foods that are high in fiber, and include plenty of fruit and vegetables (see box opposite).
- Exercise every day. Walking is helpful. If you are not able to move around or exercise, tighten and relax the muscles in your abdomen and move or lift your legs often while sitting or lying in bed.
- Try to develop a daily routine so that you have a bowel movement at the same time each day. After breakfast can be a good time for many people.
- If possible, avoid using a bedpan. Use the toilet or bedside commode.
- Discuss with your health care provider what has worked well in the past to avoid or treat constipation.
- If you are given medications to prevent constipation, take them as instructed.

EXAMPLES OF HIGH-FIBER FOODS

Oranges	Bran	Green beans	Squash
Grapefruit	Oatmeal	Cabbage	Eggplant
Melons	Figs	Brown rice	Lettuce
Prunes	Beans	Whole wheat bread	
Corn	Whole-grain cereal		Oat bran
		Kale	
Legumes (lentils, split peas)	Soybeans	Plums	
Pears	Potatoes	Mushrooms	Carrots

How to Manage Your Constipation

You can treat mild constipation with the above tips. However, if your bowels have not moved for several days, you may be at risk of severe constipation. Medications to help move your bowels may be required. Ask your health care team what they recommend.

What to Tell Your Health Care Provider If You Are Constipated

If you need to consult with your health care provider, remember to give them the following information:

1. When did you last had a bowel movement? Was it normal in size, color, and texture?

Was the stool difficult to pass?

Did you have any bleeding?

Did you have diarrhea?

2. Write down the amount and kinds of fluid and food you are drinking and eating.

3. List the names of the medications you are taking for your bowels, the amounts, and new medications or treatments since your last visit (especially if you have had an increase in pain medication).

Recipes for Regularity

Following are some tasty recipes that can keep you regular and feeling better.

Senna Tea Stewed Prunes

1 ounce (28 grams) senna leaves

1 quart water (approximately 1 liter)

1 pound (about 0.5 kilograms) prunes

Optional: Infuse with thickly sliced lemon or orange with the outer rind sliced off for more intricate flavor and aroma.

Boil the senna leaves gently in the water. Strain off the leaves and add the prunes. Continue to simmer until most of the liquid is absorbed or evaporated.

Dose: Eat 1 to 3 prunes every 2 or 3 days.

Senna tea can also be brewed with just the leaves and used to regulate bowel function.

Success Spread

¼ pound raisins
¼ pound currants
¼ pound prunes
¼ pound figs
¼ pound dates
8 ounces prune concentrate

Optional: Add a dash of cinnamon, nutmeg, or vanilla. Lemon juice is nice to cut some of the sweetness.

Put the fruit through a grinder or food processor. Blend in the prune concentrate. Store in the refrigerator. Use 2 to 3 tablespoons daily for regular action. This is a pleasant spread on toast.

1-2-3 Prune Pleasure

1 cup bran
2 cups prune juice
3 cups applesauce

Optional: Add freshly grated apples, oatmeal, and raisins, and you have Swiss muesli cereal.

Mix all together. This makes a tasty addition to hot cereals. Begin by using 2 to 4 tablespoons, and increase or decrease as needed.

DIARRHEA

Diarrhea is defined as 2 or more loose or watery stools per day. Diarrhea can be caused by both chemotherapy and radiation therapy. If you are receiving radiation therapy to an area that does not include your abdomen (stomach area), you will not get diarrhea from the radiation therapy alone. However, if you are receiving radiation treatments to your bowel area, the diarrhea can increase over time.

Tips to Slow Your Gut

- Avoid eating foods high in fiber, fatty foods, rich desserts, or other foods that increase bowel activity, such as hot peppers, coffee, alcohol, and high-fat foods.
- Use Imodium-AD or Lomotil. These are over-the-counter drugs to slow down diarrhea. Take as instructed on the label.
- If diarrhea occurs after meals, plan your activities accordingly.
- Increase your intake of liquids to ten to twelve 8-ounce glasses per day.
- Be sure to tell your health care provider you have had diarrhea.
- If following these steps does not stop your diarrhea, you should call your health care team for further advice and treatment.

Other Reasons to Call Your Health Care Provider

- You develop a temperature over 100.3°F.
- You are vomiting and not able to keep fluids down.
- You become dizzy.
- Your urine becomes dark in color.
- You have bloody stools.

PROMOTING BETTER SLEEP

A poor night's sleep can be frustrating and leave you tired and less than enthusiastic to face the day. Everyone has a bad night now and then, and these tips should keep you from forming negative sleep patterns. Try these simple steps to encourage good sleep habits.

Try to exercise daily or every other day (walking, light jogging, swimming, and bicycling are all beneficial). Exercising early in the day is best. Avoid vigorous exercise in the evening or 3 to 4 hours before you go to bed. Exercising too close to your bedtime, even easy walking, will stimulate your body and can make it harder to fall asleep.

Stick to a regular sleeping schedule for both going to bed and waking up. Consistency is key to good sleep habits. Even if your sleep is interrupted, try to get up at the same time each day. Your sleep-wake cycle is usually based on what time you get up in the morning. So, if you sleep in late one morning your sleep the next night will be affected as well. Going to bed early to get caught up on sleep is okay. Try not to go to bed more than 1 to 2 hours before your usual bedtime. Try to avoid sleeping long hours on the weekends or holidays.

If you nap, try to keep the nap between 20 and 30 minutes. Sleeping longer can disrupt your nighttime sleep. You may want to use an alarm or have someone wake you up.

Try to make sure your bedroom is quiet, well ventilated, and at a comfortable sleeping temperature (60 to 65°F). A small fan or white-noise device can cover up other sounds. Carpeting, shades, and draperies also can help a room to be more soundproof. A new mattress or adding an egg crate mattress may also be helpful.

A warm (not hot) bath before retiring can be helpful.

Turn off the lights and light a candle to create a calmer atmosphere while soaking in the tub. Light reading or sex can be relaxing, too. Other options include listening to peaceful music or mindful relaxation.

Try to avoid tobacco, caffeine, and alcohol in the evening. Instead, drink an herbal tea or warm milk before sleep. If you are hungry at bedtime, have a light snack, such as crackers, toast, fruit, or milk. Spicy foods should be avoided.

Relaxation exercises can be good to try, as you fall asleep. Tighten and relax various parts of your body and be aware of your breathing. Think of a favorite place, such as a beach or the mountains. Try to imagine the sounds you hear at that particular place so you have a strong, pleasant image in your mind.

If you are unable to sleep after a half hour or so, get up. Move to another room; avoid bright lights and any major activity. Try reading something that isn't too serious, scary, or entertaining. After about 20 minutes go back to bed. If you still can't sleep, try getting up again and read or watch TV, or try using some relaxation techniques.

Lastly, if you continue to have sleep problems, tell your health care team. There are medications that can help you get a good night's sleep.

LYMPHEDEMA

Lymphedema is swelling in an arm or leg. It is caused by blockage of the lymph nodes, usually in the armpit or groin area, from surgery or radiation. Lymphedema can occur immediately after surgery or many months and even years after cancer treatment. In addition to being visible and affecting motion, lymphedema can be painful, and can be aggravated by common everyday activities like picking up grandchildren, using a computer, washing dishes, housework, or knitting.

Signs to Report

1. Swelling in your arm, hand, foot, or leg (on the side you had surgery)
2. A feeling of fullness in the area of surgery
3. Pain or soreness in one area or that came on suddenly
4. Redness or warmth

Helpful Tips for Preventing and Managing Lymphedema

- Measure your extremity regularly so you are aware of any changes. It is important to intervene early to minimize the swelling.
- Elevate the swollen extremity at least 20 minutes 3 to 4 times a day.
- Use exercise, self-massage, and gentle stretching to move the fluid toward the body, which we think may help new channels develop for the lymph fluid to drain. Do this at least twice a day.
- Avoid heavy lifting on your affected side. Work within your comfort limits. Don't strain to lift heavy shopping bags. If you want to be able to lift heavier items, you need to strengthen your arm

gradually and work up to carrying heavier loads.

- Keep your skin moist and free of cuts and cracks.
- If you develop signs of an infection (redness, warmth, inflammation, or red streaks) call your health care provider.
- Report changes in sensation, pain, numbness, or tightness of clothing, watches, bracelets, or rings.
- Wear a professionally fitted compression sleeve or stocking, and if necessary learn to bandage the extremity during flares.
- Exercise is helpful in reducing and controlling lymphedema. After surgery, gentle stretching and range-of-motion exercise should be started. Over time, regular activities and exercise should be resumed. We don't understand the exact mechanisms of lymphedema, but we think that the muscle contractions of exercise help to move the excess fluid out of the limb.

PERIPHERAL NEUROPATHY

Peripheral neuropathy is a loss of sensation that usually occurs in the fingers, hands, toes, and feet. Certain types of chemotherapy (vincristine, paclitaxel, and cisplatin) and tumors can injure the peripheral nerves, causing numbness and tingling in the hands and feet, muscle pain, and sensitivity to touch. In extreme cases, peripheral neuropathy can impair walking and balance. Peripheral neuropathy can interfere with daily activities, such as dressing, eating, and walking. Although there is no way to prevent peripheral neuropathy completely, it is important to pay attention to the early signs, such as changes in sensation in your fingers and toes, so that further damage can be prevented, if possible.

LONG-TERM SIDE EFFECTS OF TREATMENT AND CANCER

Osteoporosis

As if cancer and its treatment aren't enough, we are learning that osteoporosis is a side effect of many cancer treatments. Osteoporosis is a thinning of the bones that makes them more porous, brittle, and susceptible to fracture. Bone loss occurs during treatment and is a silent, asymptomatic side effect. Although both men and women lose bone when receiving chemotherapeutic agents, such as doxorubicin and methotrexate, and steroids, such as prednisone or Decadron, the effects of these bone-wasting drugs are greatest on premenopausal women, who often lose ovarian function and go through early menopause as yet another unpleasant and distressing side effect of chemotherapy. Studies comparing the bone loss of premenopausal women and postmenopausal women demonstrate that women who are premenopausal before treatment and are thrown into menopause during or following treatment lose a remarkable amount of bone. The question remains unanswered about how much bone is regained after treatment ends and how the structure of the bone is ultimately affected. We know that during the first five years of menopause women typically lose 2 to 5 percent of their bone density a year. So, when the loss of bone density during chemotherapy is added to the normal equation, these prematurely menopausal young women have lost a lot of bone and are at a much higher risk of fracturing a bone and suffering the painful consequences.

I don't want it to sound as though postmenopausal women, and men, are not at risk for bone loss. They are. Bone loss is related to chemotherapy and inactivity, and cancer treatment increases bone loss, which means that men lose bone mass at a younger age and postmenopausal women have accelerated bone loss. Although there are medications to prevent bone loss and rebuild bone density, prevention of the bone loss is of utmost importance.

There are many risk factors for osteoporosis. Physical factors that predispose us to osteoporosis include being female, having a family history of osteoporosis, being tall or thin (less than 18 percent body fat), being fair skinned, or having a history of clinical depression, thyroid disease, and premature menopause. Although we have little control over the physical factors that put us at risk for osteoporosis, we can modify our lifestyle risks.

Behavioral or lifestyle factors that further increase the risk of osteoporosis include a history of smoking, living a sedentary lifestyle, or exercising too vigorously. High levels of vigorous exercise can cause amenorrhea (no menstrual periods) and low estrogen levels. The excess consumption of caffeine (more than about 2 cups of coffee per day) contributes to bone loss by increasing the excretion of calcium. Unfortunately, the more caffeine you drink, the more calcium your body loses. Drinking much more than about two and a half 4-ounce glasses of wine or 12-ounce glasses of beer per day interferes with the bone's ability to rebuild old bone and lay down new bone. If your liver is overstressed because of a somewhat overindulgent lifestyle or damage from medications that can be harmful to your bone health, too, the production and metabolism of estrogen, which is important for bone health and growth, is impaired. Although it is difficult to change our usual ways, we can consciously make decisions to change our daily habits to increase our physical activity levels and dietary intake of calcium and vitamin D and decrease caffeine and alcohol intake.

Medications to keep us healthy or treat cancer can also cause bone loss. These include drugs, such as steroids (e.g., prednisone or Decadron) for treatment of your cancer or such diseases as asthma; the regular use of anticonvulsant medications, such as diazepam (Valium) or lorazepam (Ativan); and some chemotherapeutic agents, such as doxorubicin (Adriamycin) and methotrexate, used to treat many different cancers.

Heart Disease

Many cancer treatments cause weight gain, and that combined with the well-meaning advice of health care providers to rest, and the effect of some drugs on the heart, is the perfect formula for heart disease. Research has demonstrated the relationship between excess weight, obesity, inactivity, and diets high in fat and the subsequent development of heart disease. Statisticians have developed models that suggest that cancer survivors are four times more likely to die from a heart attack than their "healthy cancer-free" counterparts. Although no studies have been conducted that look specifically at the effects of exercise on preventing heart disease in cancer patients, our understanding of the mechanisms of heart disease strongly suggests that exercise is beneficial. Exercise in cancer patients and healthy persons helps with weight loss and reduction of blood pressure and lipid levels (e.g., triglycerides and cholesterol) and strengthens the heart muscle to pump more efficiently with less effort. With the risk factors of weight gain, inactivity, chemotherapy, and other common cardiovascular problems, such as high blood pressure and high cholesterol levels, it only makes sense to modify your lifestyle by increasing your physical activity level to ward off some of these threats to your well-being.

SUMMARY

Exercise isn't a panacea for every side effect you may experience during treatment, but it does dramatically improve quality of life and can prevent some of the long-term side effects of treatment. The sooner you become in tune with your body and learn to recognize and manage your side effects and symptoms, you will not only feel better but be able to do more of the things in life that you value and that are important to you. If your side effects persist despite your aggressive attempts to control them, talk to your health care team and describe what is happening. Don't wait until your next appointment—ask for help now; simply changing, adding, or deleting a medication or learning another self-management technique may be all you need to feel better today. Your quality of life is important, and you can't enjoy it when you feel bad!

KEY POINTS

- Learn to manage your side effects early in your treatment.
- If your management techniques are not working as well as you would like, work with your health care team to develop a better plan.
- Manage your side effects early before they get bad. This is especially true of pain and nausea—take your medication regularly, as prescribed.
- Know that your side effects can be managed. Ask for help if you aren't feeling well.
- Drink an adequate amount of fluids (e.g., water or juice).
- If your side effects are not controlled, it is difficult to exercise.

CHAPTER 4

SETTING GOALS
FOR A LIFETIME OF EXERCISE

The most common complaint I hear is, "I'm too tired to exercise!" Or, "I'm too busy, how could I possibly make time to exercise?" Fatigue is an overwhelming and all too common side effect of cancer treatments, but it is not a reason, or even an excuse, to avoid exercise. In fact, most of my patients tell me that the most important time to exercise is when they feel their worst. Now this may not be intuitively obvious, but expending energy (in reasonable amounts) builds new energy. When you are tired and you make yourself move, you get energy back and feel better.

Starting an exercise program is a challenge for anyone, let alone when you are confronted with or recovering from cancer treatment. What most commonly stops us from achieving our goals? Excuses. We use excuses to hide our self-imposed limitations and our fear of failure, which are our greatest barriers to success in anything we seek to achieve, not just exercise. So, we make up excuses with which we are more or less comfortable, and they become our barriers to achieving our goals.

To stay focused on your goal, which I recommend to all my patients, keep a record or a log of exercise. Record the type of exercise you did, how long you did it for, how hard you exercised on the RPE (see Chapter 5) scale, and how you felt during and after the exercise. An entry in your log can be completed in about one minute and will provide a wealth of information to help guide and motivate you to exercise. If you did not exercise, record why you missed your exercise session. Not only will you see your progress, but you will be able to identify your excuses and barriers to exercise.

Now is the time to assess what keeps you from succeeding at exercise. What are your personal traps and self-defeating behaviors? For most people it is not that they do not understand the benefits of exercise, it is that they are afraid, afraid of starting something new and not succeeding. Confront that fear. A major obstacle to living to our full potential is a belief that we cannot achieve or succeed in reaching our personal goals. Often that fear keeps us from even trying.

Rely on your inner strength to overcome and change your old ways and to exceed your self-imposed limitations and expectations. Forget what others may be thinking about you. Who cares? Be willing to do what is really important to you, in your heart. Free yourself of the old ways that limit you and your ability to embrace life fully and see life as a wonderful adventure.

HAVE A GOAL

A goal gives us a purpose and a reason to get up and exercise. Choose an event in the next two to four months, and focus your exercise on that goal. For some people the goal may be to walk out of the hospital, walk around the park with your walking group, or walk in a local cancer fund-raising event. Whatever your goal, make it realistic and achievable. Having a buddy, dog, or other companion to exercise with helps to keep you on a regular schedule, and a log helps you to see how you are progressing.

Janice was a 38-year-old single mother of two children when she was diagnosed with lymphoma. She remembers the doctor telling her she had lymphoma and then couldn't hear any more, terrified for her children and her future. Fortunately, Sarah, her younger sister, was there to hear and later relate the details of treatment for Janice. When Janice started treatment she was afraid and certain she would not be able to function.

The following is Janice's description of the effects of exercise on her mood, attitude, and general outlook on life. "I was angry and spent most days on the couch feeling depressed and sorry for myself. I didn't deserve this [cancer]. When my sister pushed me to sign up for the Cancer Fitness program, I was skeptical and lacked motivation. However, very quickly I could see that each day I got a little more confident, because I could see that I was actually moving toward my goal. At the end of week 2, I could see changes in my attitude and outlook, and I was starting to feel strong again. Knowing that I'm still capable of accomplishing my goals gave me confidence and restored my feelings of hope. Now I feel like each day is a gift to enjoy and cherish."

A QUESTION OF COMMITMENT

Write down your answers to these questions: Have you made a decision to exercise? What are your reasons for exercise? Can you commit to exercising 10 to 30 minutes at least three days this week? Can you see yourself beginning an exercise program? Can you see yourself sticking to the program? What will stop you from succeeding? What are your personal barriers? What are your fears? What are the excuses you might use to quit the exercise program? Some common examples are feeling bad from exercise, exercising alone, and feeling embarrassed or self-conscious. What do you need to stay with your program? Many people need an exercise companion or a safe place to exercise where they won't feel embarrassed or uncomfortable about their bodies, and some people find that joining a group helps them to stay with an exercise routine. Once you have examined your reasons for beginning the Cancer Fitness program and identified some of your obstacles to success, we can actually start examining ways to handle the barriers that may keep you from succeeding in reaching your exercise and life goals.

TIPS FOR EXERCISE SUCCESS

There's no doubt that starting an exercise program is a challenge, especially when you are beginning or in the midst of cancer treatment or if you have had unpleasant or unsuccessful experiences with exercise. For many people, however, the diagnosis of cancer is the call to take charge of your life. Often, I think, our lifestyle changes are motivated by fear of death or disability or a strong desire to be there for loved ones. My patient, Lori, started exercising the day she learned that her mammogram showed a highly suspicious mass. She hasn't stopped exercising since and proclaims that the exercise she did before her surgery made the recovery much easier. Lori now advises anyone she knows to start exercising before they being their treatments and to find a friend to exercise with. The following are some tips that Lori and many of my other patients have found helpful in successfully integrating a consistent exercise program into their lives.

- Review the benefits of exercise. If you understand how you will benefit from exercise you will be more motivated to exercise. And, the more you benefit, the more motivated you will become. Your benefits from consistent exercise will be rewarding, and for many people, that's the very motivation they need to keep exercising.
- Write down all of your personal reasons for exercising. Over the next few days write every reason you can think of. Keep the list in a visible place, like on your refrigerator or your bathroom mirror, so you can review it regularly. Some examples are:

  —feel better during my cancer treatment
  —recover more quickly from my surgery and treatment
  —have more energy for family
  —be able to fit into all the clothes in my closet
  —be able to live a long, healthy life
  —feel more comfortable when I go out in public
  —be able to climb stairs without getting so breathless

Having a list is important. When your enthusiasm is waning, review all the reasons you decided to exercise consistently and I think you will feel motivated again. I've seen this simple tip work well for hundreds of patients.

- Dedicate a time for exercise. I find that people are most successful if they exercise first thing in the morning or dedicate their lunch hour to exercise. Once you reserve your special time for exercise, protect the time and make it a priority. This will help to make exercise more easily become a lifelong habit. If you leave exercise until later in the day, it's too easy for other things to get in the way, like running errands or picking up the kids or getting stuck in traffic.

- Be accountable. Find a buddy to exercise with. Research shows that people who exercise with a friend or a group are more successful at consistently sticking to a program. Knowing you have to be at the street corner at 7 A.M. to meet a friend to walk with is great motivation to show up. After all, they are relying on you. Many people have told me that they are most successful in exercise if they involve their families, which also has the benefit of teaching children or grandchildren the values of exercise. What helps me? My dog. Rain or shine, Max relies on me and holds me accountable for our daily activity. He never fails to remind me if I'm late or, heaven forbid, if we miss our daily outing! Dogs are terrific exercise companions.

- Have goals—a long-term goal and lots of short-term goals. Each time you reach one of your goals, celebrate. It feels good to reach your goals. Each time you successfully accomplish your goal you are one step closer to being transformed into a regular exerciser.

- Reward yourself when you meet your goals. Ron told me that each time he meets his monthly exercise goals he goes to the movies. Sally from Seattle rewards herself by putting $2 in a piggy bank at the end of a successful week of exercise. With the reward money she treats herself to something she wouldn't usually buy herself.

- Keep a log of your exercise. Keep track of how long you exercised and what you did. After a few weeks calculate your weekly total exercise time. I think you'll surprise yourself.

- Make exercise fun. Join a group of friends, take your dog, or go to a special place to exercise when you have time. If you like to exercise to music, use a headset, or if you're inside play some music or set up the television in a location where you can easily see it. If you prefer the quiet and solitude of exercise, go it alone. Do whatever makes exercise most enjoyable. If exercise is fun you'll be more likely to follow your program consistently.

- Avoid injury by wearing good shoes and comfortable clothing.

- See your results, and enjoy getting compliments for your achievements. For some people, the compliments and encouragement of friends is the best motivation of all.

GREEN LIGHT

You should begin by congratulating yourself. By reading this book you are taking the first steps to strengthening your body and mind and healing from your cancer. The process of transforming or improving your strength requires persistence and determination. Become familiar with the common barriers that change the green light (I'm doing great in my exercise program) to a red light (the excuses that stop your exercise program). There will be highs and lows and many plateaus and perhaps even unexpected challenges from your treatments, but don't let impatience or frustration prevent you from continuing in your quest for better physical and mental health. Keep looking for the green light, and don't let anything stop you from moving forward despite frustration or other barriers. Confront your excuses and barriers to exercise by creating your own barrier-busting plan.

Perhaps you have just started the Cancer Fitness program and you've had a terrifically successful three weeks. You feel like your body, mind, and spirit are one, and that you can, for the first time in your life, succeed at an exercise program. But around the corner is the red light, a barrier you hadn't expected. What is your plan to handle the unexpected? Follow the suggestions in the next few sections of this chapter to create a plan to keep you on track to reach your short-term and long-term goals and keep the green light glowing.

BARRIER BUSTING

Begin by developing a barrier-busting plan. These three questions should be thought through carefully.

What to do?

Think about your exercise plan and goals for the week. Are they reasonable and achievable? What may get in the way of reaching your goals? How will you handle the obstacles that get in the way? Make a list of all the potential barriers and excuses you can think of. Make goals that you can achieve. Remember, your first goal is success!

Why do it?

After you have thought about your activities for the week, think about why you are following this plan. Why are you committed to this program? What is your backup plans if you do not achieve your goals? How will you modify your future goals if you do not attain your goals for the week? Maybe you were a little too ambitious in your goals for the first week of the program. Take a look at what you did do. How did you feel? Were you pushing too hard to achieve what you did this week? Honestly evaluate your exercise for the week, and then revise your goals for next week so that they are achievable. It's hard to know reasonable goals for yourself when you first start to exercise, and even if you are a regular exerciser, cancer treatments can quickly change your endurance and strength. So, don't be hard on yourself for not reaching your goals, just sit down and reevaluate your next goals so that you will succeed.

How did it go?

At the end of the week, evaluate the effectiveness of your plan. Did you achieve what you set out to do? Were your goals reasonable? If you did not completely achieve your goals, rework your plan for the next week. There is nothing wrong with changing your goals. It's the smart thing to do, particularly if you had difficulty attaining your goals the previous week. By being honest with yourself about what you can truly achieve, you will be able to establish a successful exercise regimen and one that can be enjoyable.

Achieving your goals helps you to dream of bigger goals and become inspired to reach a little further. Confronting your personal obstacles to success in exercise and life creates optimism, which helps you to look toward the future. Laurel was 59 years old when she started the Cancer Fitness program. She was nearing the end of a difficult chemotherapy treatment for colon cancer, and here she describes her experience with exercise:

> The physical and emotional changes that occurred in just the first few weeks were inspiring. I examined my obstacles (never succeeding before with exercise, being too tired, having too much to do) and posted them on the refrigerator next to my goals and my list of reasons to exercise. Every day I reviewed them and then one day I realized I was reaching goals that I never thought I could.

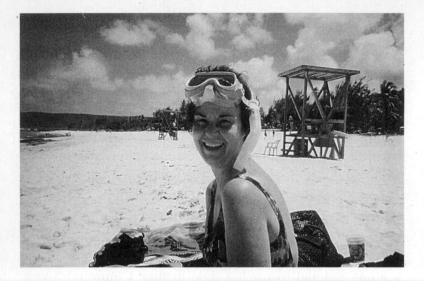

Make your exercise fun. This is the happy face of a woman who is going snorkeling for the first time ever.

MOVEMENT IS EXERCISE

All too often we fail to realize that when we move our bodies, whether it is pushing a grocery cart, walking up a flight of stairs, or running through the woods, we are getting exercise. Many people set themselves up to fail because they think that they need to do a certain type of exercise and that it has to be unpleasant. Actually, very modest exercise that is done consistently can give you incredible benefits. There's a catch, however: you have to do the exercise regularly. You need to make it part of your life, whether you walk up the stairs instead of taking the elevator or park at the outer edge of the parking lot so that you have a greater distance to walk to your office or into the mall. Our daily movements add up, and the more movement we do the stronger and healthier our bodies become. Keep your goals reasonable and attainable.

REASSESSING ONE'S GOALS

Grant was a 77-year-old former coal miner who had developed lung cancer. Grant's goal to himself was to have energy to walk up the two flights of stairs to his apartment at least once every day instead of taking the elevator. When he first set this goal Grant didn't realize how debilitated he had become, and he struggled, having to sit to rest several times, to make it up the first flight of stairs. So, Grant revised his goal and decided that for the next three weeks he would walk up one flight of stairs at least once a day. Being a stubborn and determined guy, he started adding a little more each week, so that by the end of the three weeks, he was actually climbing the stairs two times a day, and on occasions when he had a lot of energy, three times a day. By breaking his exercise into smaller pieces, he was able to reach his goal, and at the end of three weeks he climbed up the two flights of stairs to his apartment, slowly, but succeeded in climbing them without stopping to rest.

SETTING GOALS

We all need strategies to maintain our efforts in the face of setbacks, slumps, and so on. Setting goals is a simple way to stay motivated and focused on your exercise program. Success in achieving your goals is dependent on setting reasonable and attainable goals. We are motivated by our goals, but we must set our own goals and choose what is best for us. Goal setting is fundamental not only to successful exercise habits but also for pursuing a productive and meaningful life. Without a goal and a plan in exercise and life, we tend to wander and things do not get done, or at least not as efficiently as they could. Goal setting provides a directed course of action, like a blueprint, for your athletic goals as well as attainment of other life pursuits.

You need to ask yourself several questions. Why is it important to you to achieve this goal? How long have you wanted to achieve this goal? What have you done to achieve your goal? Is the goal realistic? What are the steps you need to take to achieve your goal? This last question should help you to break your goals into smaller steps that you can successfully achieve. As the steps build so will your confidence and ability.

Goals must be your own, not what someone else thinks would be good for you. You must want to attain your goal and feel committed. Several actions can help you become committed to attaining your goals. First, set reasonable goals and make the commitment to attain them by talking to friends and family. Increase the probability of your success by making a "public" statement and commitment. By openly stating what you are working toward, your friends and family will be able to support you in meeting those goals. They may want to know how you are progressing and may even want to join you in your exercise session. Often, if you tell people what your goal is—for example, to walk in the local cancer fundraiser or complete a 50-mile bike ride—your friends will want to support and help you to succeed. The strength you get from telling people about your goals will help you to push through on days when you are tired or not feeling your best.

There are always those people who consciously or unconsciously try to sabotage our plans. Some caring family and friends won't want you to exercise because they worry you could hurt yourself or that it may be dangerous for someone with cancer, or they may even be jealous that you have the energy, discipline, and commitment to make a lifestyle change. It's easy to say, "stay away from these people," but if this person is your spouse or best friend, there's trouble. Often the idea of change is threatening, and simply by talking with them about why becoming more physically active is important to you and your health may be sufficient to allay their fears or concerns. When people understand that exercise is safe and learn the potential health benefits, their attitudes often change and they become supportive cheerleaders.

Writing your goals down also helps to stay focused and motivated. By writing your goals down you become clearer in the steps that are needed to attain them and how you will go about getting there. If you maintain a regular journal or log of your exercise you can clearly see your progress toward attainment. This in itself is motivating.

HAVE A PLAN

Jerry was 63 years old when he was diagnosed with lung cancer. Ever since his youthful days in the navy, Jerry took great pleasure in smoking. He enjoyed the taste, the way the cigarette felt in his fingers, and the smoke as it curled up past his nose. That is, until he was diagnosed with lung cancer. After a long surgery, Jerry vowed he would stop smoking, which he did—cold turkey. He was proud to be able to quit so abruptly, but after a few weeks of not smoking he started feeling down and out of sorts. Jerry's wife, Rosie, realized he was feeling blue and irritable from both the chemotherapy treatments and smoking. She suggested they start to walk together to get out of the house. It was spring, and Rosie thought getting out in the fresh air would cheer him up. Jerry liked the idea, and they enjoyed their times together and made an effort to walk after meals—his favorite time to smoke. Rosie and Jerry both struggled with making exercise a regular part of their lives. They didn't know how to gauge when they had gone too far or how to pace themselves. On one occasion they walked so far that Jerry couldn't make it home and had to ride the bus. On other occasions they walked so far that when they finally got home Jerry had to sleep and was too exhausted to exercise or do anything else for many days. When we met, I suggested they make an exercise plan with weekly goals. Rosie liked the idea and Jerry didn't oppose it, as long as Rosie made the plan Jerry was worn out from pushing too hard. So, Rosie and I worked out a gradual and progressive exercise plan. Several weeks later Jerry said, "When Rosie and I have goals and a plan, exercise is okay. Actually, it was a breakthrough. Exercise got me out of depression and helped me to believe in myself, face the challenge of lung cancer, and accept my life voyage as a stronger person both physically and emotionally."

KEEPING A LOG

I generally suggest that you keep a simple record of what you did, where you exercised, what the weather was like, how long and how hard you exercised, and how you felt. Some folks like to grade their performance from A—you felt great and had an outstanding workout—to F—failing to meet your goal or not feeling well. If you use the grading system, I suggest that when you are having a C day, cut back the intensity of your workout. Go easier and maybe less distance and time. If the next day you still feel like you are a C, cut the workout in half. On days that are a D or F, I strongly suggest you skip the workout and rest. This doesn't mean standing on your feet or substituting your exercise program for other chores; this means reading, playing or working at the computer, or watching a movie—doing restful activities. If you start to have a bunch of D and F days, well, I suspect you need to have an honest talk with the little voices in your head. Are you really all that tired, are you getting sick or overtrained, or are you simply using the grading scale as another excuse to skip your daily exercise?

Here is what a few sample entries in an exercise log might look like (see Chapter 5 for an explanation of RPE):

Date: 7/23/01 **Time:** 5 P.M. **Weather:** 89° humid and cloudy

Place: Home loop by the park 3/4 mile

Activity: Walked 3 minutes to warm up. Alternated walking and trotting for 7 minutes. Walked home last 2 minutes.

Time: 12 minutes

RPE: 13

Grade: B+. Felt too hot to push myself. Need to drink more water before and during exercise.

Date: 7/25/01 **Time:** 8 A.M. **Weather:** 68° sunny and no wind
Place: Horse farm loop 43 miles
Activity: Cycled with the group. Steady pace except hard effort up Camel Hill, but no camels at the top today.
Time: 3 hours
RPE: 14
Grade: A. Felt great. Legs rested. Able to push the pace today.

Date: 7/26/01 **Time:** 8 A.M. **Weather:** Inside about 74°
Place: At home
Activity: Resistance Exercise Program A
Leg extension: Black band 3 sets of 8 reps
Biceps curls: Red band 3 sets of 12 reps; too easy
Side leg kicks: Blue band 3 sets of 8; tough!
Overhead pull-downs: Blue band 3 sets of 10 reps
Squats: Black band 3 sets of 8; hard
Pectoral press: Red band 3 sets of 9 reps
Curl-ups (abdominals): about 50 lost count
Curl-ups (abdominals): about 50 lost count
Time: 31 minutes
RPE: 14 to 15
Grade: A. Felt great. Really getting stronger. Need to increase resistance band on biceps curls.

Some people prefer to record their aerobic exercise in a log that is in a calendar format. An example of what a calendar exercise log might look like follows.

1	2	3	4	5	6	7
walk 15 minutes; RPE 12: grade B feel like I'm dragging	rest day	walk 20 minutes; 3 minutes at fast pace; RPE 12 to 14; grade A	rest day	30 minute walk at steady pace; RPE 13; grade A feel great	rest day	group walk for 30 minutes; moderate pace; RPE 13; grade A-

8	9	10	11	12	13	14
rest day	walk 20 minutes with 3x 2 minutes at a fast pace; RPE 13 to 15; grade A++	Rest day chemo treatment	Rest day to recover from treatment	Walk 10 minutes easy pace; RPE 12; grade B+ felt better after walk	Walked 15 minutes at moderated pace; RPE 13; grade A-	Rest day feel really good.

Some people find a day-by-day record of their resistance exercises is helpful (see page 105). You can see what weights of resistance band you used last time you exercised, and you can see your progress. The exercise log here is an example of a resistance exercise log for the Cancer Fitness resistance exercise program. You can tailor a log like this to the specific exercises you do, if they differ from the Cancer Fitness program.

What I find most helpful with an exercise log is that you can see your improvement over time. This is the best positive feedback in the world. The log is also a terrific way to understand why you may not be feeling as sharp as you did a few weeks ago: have you increased your exercise time, distance, or intensity? Are your "grades" going down? Is there a trend in your log to suggest that you might be getting rundown or overtrained? You can see all these things in your logs, if you are honest and diligent in writing down your exercise experiences.

Personally, I like to write things in my log like "stopped to watch sandhill cranes roosting in Jim's field" or "hard steady climb to top of Teton Pass (8,400 feet), sweet smell of pine and cold wind blowing over the old snow pack at the summit. Exhilarating descent back into the valley." When I include special places where I go for a run or walk, my log becomes a diary of my travels and life adventures that I enjoy looking back on, and a wonderful way to remember special times with family or friends hiking, biking, and sometimes just being together on a recovery day.

RESISTANCE EXERCISE A

Exercises	Date			Date			Date	
	Reps+Sets	Band Color/Wt		Reps+Sets	Band Color/Wt		Reps+Sets	Band Color/Wt
Squats								
Lat pull-downs								
Leg extension								
Flies								
Hip adduction								
Bicep curls								
Hip abduction								

MAKE A COMMITMENT
TO YOURSELF

When you decide to start your own exercise program, make a promise to yourself that you will commit to start and follow a program for at least 12 weeks. Do not let yourself down.

Then look back again at your barrier-busting plan and determine how and what will help you to stay right on track—keep the green light glowing. It's easy to quit—a lot easier than finding the self-discipline to commit to improving your health through exercise. Consistent exercise is one of the most important promises you ever make to yourself.

Some people find they can keep their promise better if they have a contract with themselves—such as the one on the opposite page—to exercise for 12 weeks. If signing a contract and then hanging it on your bathroom mirror or on the refrigerator will help you to keep your promise, then use this tool.

Make the vow to exercise, give it a try, and then see how much you change—both physically and emotionally. If you can commit to 12 weeks of exercise, you will then be ready for the next commitment—making exercise and physical activity a regular part of your life—a choice that will bring you many rewarding health and life benefits in the years to come.

CANCER FITNESS CONTRACT

I,——————, have agreed to dutifully follow the Cancer Fitness exercise program for 12 weeks. I will begin by making a complete list of the reasons I want to start this program and all the possible barriers and excuses that I think I might encounter along the way. I will strive to make reasonable and achievable weekly goals and keep a record of my exercise accomplishments in an exercise log. I know that if I set unreasonable goals I will not succeed, but that I can revise my goals to make them realistic. I willingly acknowledge that there may be obstacles to my progress that may present a challenge that may necessitate revising my goals but that these challenges will not prevent me from completing the program.

I sign this contract today with my friend and/or exercise companion, who is my witness.

_____

Signed

_____

Date

_____

Printed Name

_____

Friend/Exercise Companion/Witness

SUMMARY

Many of my patients don't realize what an inspiration they are to other patients and people. Seeing other people like themselves who are also confronting the challenge of cancer and starting an exercise program, is an inspiration to others that they too can take charge and change their lives. It takes courage and determination to change old habits and make a personal commitment to exercise and a healthy lifestyle, but you have the courage and determination to achieve your goals. Be steadfast in your thinking and determined, like my 21-year-old friend Adam, who was diagnosed with metastatic testicular cancer and confronted the challenge and learned much more:

> I have faced death and know it's not my time. The Cancer Fitness program helped me regain my strength and get stronger than I have ever been before. Not just physically stronger, but emotionally. It has helped me get through a life transformation.

KEY POINTS

- Starting an exercise program takes commitment and determination, but the rewards will be there for you.
- Examine your barriers and excuses to exercise, and make a plan to succeed.
- Set your own goals that are reasonable and achievable.

- Keep a log of your exercise regimen so you can monitor your progress.
- Sign a contract and make a commitment to yourself to follow the Cancer Fitness program for 12 weeks, and see how it changes you physically and emotionally.

CHAPTER 5

CANCER FITNESS FUNDAMENTALS

You now have an overview of the many benefits that you can gain from an exercise program. Most Americans don't exercise. Why? Because they find exercise aversive, uncomfortable, and time-consuming. Many people think of exercise as an activity that will make them feel uncomfortable, tired, and sweaty. I don't want you to experience discomfort. Exercise should be fun and physically and emotionally restorative. I am going to introduce a different approach to exercise that will gradually bring your fitness to a level such that whether you are in the hospital, home recovering from your cancer treatment, were an inactive person or an athlete before your cancer diagnosis, you can easily incorporate it into your everyday life. First, let's review the components of an exercise program.

COMPONENTS OF EXERCISE

Although cancer and exercise research is still in an early phase, the science is rapidly moving forward, in part because of the tremendous foundation of existing research in exercise and heart disease. Basic principles about exercise intensity and duration and types of exercise give cancer researchers a solid base to move this research forward without having to do extensive studies that would repeat much of the early work scientists have already conducted on patients with heart disease and other illnesses.

An exercise prescription consists of four components:

1. type of exercise
2. frequency (how often you exercise)
3. intensity (how hard you exercise)
4. duration (how much time you exercise)

Type of exercise can be *aerobic,* which is a sustained rhythmic activity that requires oxygen for energy (e.g., walking), or *anaerobic,* short high-intensity exercise that uses energy sources not requiring oxygen (e.g., sprinting to catch a bus). *Resistance* exercise (weight lifting) can be either aerobic or anaerobic, depending on how the exercises are performed.

Frequency is how often you exercise. This component of exercise is important because it is the regularity and consistency of exercise that is key to improving your cancer-related side effects, such as fatigue, and improving your overall long-term health. How long and how often do I have to exercise? These are the two most frequently asked questions. The answer is, it varies, but science is showing us that at least 30 minutes of exercise 5 days a week is optimal for overall health—but certainly not when you first start! If you are just trying to get your leg strength and physical function back and resume a normal life, exercising 3 to 4 days a week is enough to see rapid changes in your endurance and strength. If your goal is to be competitive or complete an event that requires more endurance and strength than is needed for everyday life activities, then you may want to build up to exercising 5 days a week, but simply being more active and doing such things as walking up the stairs instead of taking the elevator will produce healthful benefits and fitness gains.

Intensity is how hard you exercise, and as I will show you, a high-intensity program is not necessary to see improvements in your fitness. *Intensity* of exercise is generally referred to as low, moderate, high, or strenuous. Some authors and many exercise trainers recommend monitoring your heart rate to determine your exercise intensity by using relatively inexpensive heart rate monitors. However, for many people who are starting exercise for the first time or who simply want to have a more active lifestyle, these devices can distract a person with confusing data. Heart rate information allows you to train scientifically at different heart rate levels, which correspond to different exercise intensities, but the data can be highly variable if you are receiving treatment. Your heart rate can also be influenced by caffeine, alcohol, medication, stress, and illness. Heart rate monitoring also can take the simple joy out of exercise for many people, who feel they now have to concentrate and decipher what the monitor is telling them.

An easy way to monitor your exercise intensity is the Borg rating of perceived exertion (RPE), a well-tested and easy way to determine how hard you are exercising. You simply rate your level of exertion or how hard you are working on a scale of 6 "no exertion" at all, to 20 "maximal exertion," as shown in Table 1.

Table 1. Borg's Rating of Perceived Exertion Scale (RPE)1

6	No exertion at all
7	Extremely light
8	
9	Very light
10	
11	Light
12	
14	Somewhat hard
15	Hard (heavy)
16	
17	Very hard
18	
19	Extremely hard
20	Maximal exertion

For correct usage of the scale the user must go to the instruction and administration given by Borg (see Borg G. *Borg's Perceived Exercise and Pain Scales*. Champaign. IL: Human Kinetics Books, 1998) or to the folder published by Borg on the RPE scale.

For this system to be effective, you must learn to listen to your body and determine how hard you are breathing and how hard you feel you are exercising. If you are just beginning an exercise program, your target RPE should be between 11 (easy walking or exercising and can talk comfortably) and 14 (brisk walking or exercising at an intensity where you are breathing harder but can still talk), so that you are not feeling uncomfortable and can begin to increase the amount of time you are able to move around. As you become stronger your target should be to exercise at an RPE between 13 and 15.

Science has shown us that exercising at an RPE of 13 to 15 is closely equivalent to exercising at a heart rate that is 60 to 80 percent of your maximum heart rate, the range that is optimal for improving cardiovascular fitness and health. If your goal is to start training for a particular event or competition, then I recommend heart rate–based training, but if you are simply interested in improving your health and increasing your activity level, then this method of rating your effort and intensity will be sufficient and allow your mind to be free.

LOW-, MODERATE-, AND HIGH-INTENSITY EXERCISE

Low-intensity physical activities include slow walking (less than 2 mph), sitting at the computer, watching television, or playing cards. All are activities that don't raise your heart rate, make you sweaty, or help your current and future health. Activities that promote health require you to move more and

will increase your heart rate and breathing rate, but not necessarily to an uncomfortable degree.

Such activities as brisk walking, bicycling, and swimming
constitute moderate activity and can have a beneficial effect
on your tolerance for treatment and your health in the
future. Moderate activity is the type of activity I recommend.
Activities that are easy to incorporate into your daily routine
are those you will stick to for life, which is why I generally
suggest that most people start with walking. It is important
for you to exercise during treatment, but it is the lifelong
adoption of a more active lifestyle that will keep you healthy
long into the future.

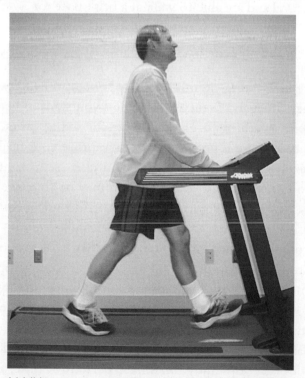

Walking on a treadmill during one of the studies.

The aversive exercise that most people think of when I suggest an exercise program is high intensity. This type of exercise makes your heart pound, your breathing labored, and your body sweaty. High-intensity exercise is the type of exercise that makes many people want to avoid exercise entirely, not the increase in heart rate that you may feel walking up a flight of stairs. Even people who don't exercise can remember having pushed themselves too hard, not feeling good during the activity, and feeling exhausted afterward—and often this is why they don't want or like to exercise. You want to avoid this. Go slowly, and build up to a moderate pace. If it hurts or makes you feel bad, slow down! Once you sustain a baseline fitness level and are able to walk at a brisk pace for 30 minutes uninterrupted, then you may want to consider increasing your speed or selecting a more challenging route with more hills. If you spend a brief amount of time—seconds to a few minutes—working at this increased intensity, you will get stronger, fitter, and faster. Again, unless you want to become a competitive athlete or are training for a big event, high-intensity exercise is not necessary to improve your health.

Duration, or how much time you exercise, is something that you must increase gradually. You may be able to exercise 5 days a week or every other day, but I do not recommend exercising more than 30 minutes at first, unless you are in good physical condition to start with. My goal for you is to learn to enjoy movement and activity. For some people this may mean exercising for 2 minutes in the morning by walking around the house or to the end of hospital ward and then repeating the activity two or three times during the day. By gradually building a fitness base, you will be able to do more activities that you enjoy for longer periods of time, and not become so worn out.

My research has shown that during chemotherapy, 10 to 20 minutes of exercise done all at once or broken into short sessions has a profound effect on reducing fatigue while increasing fitness. Patients who exercise every day for short periods of time (10 to 20 minutes) experience the best effects of exercise, but those people who exercise every other day are still able to enjoy substantial declines in fatigue, improvements in quality of life, and fitness during chemotherapy. For most people, 10 to 30 minutes of exercise is a reasonable and achievable goal and one that can be fit into your daily routine.

CHILDHOOD MEMORIES

Exercise for many people is not fun. You may have unpleasant memories of pushing yourself too hard or not being able to keep up, or perhaps even being made fun of by other children. Jack had similar memories. He was a self-assured, chief executive officer of a large company and had recently been diagnosed with chronic myelogenous leukemia. Jack was an ambitious man, and his biggest concern was being able to continue working and leading his company. I approached Jack about exercise, and he looked at me, shook his head, and said, "I can't exercise." I was truly surprised by his answer, given his air of confidence, and replied, "Why, anyone can exercise, it's just moving around. You 'exercised' when you walked in here." Jack was taken aback by my response but still shook his head and said, "No, everyone has to walk or crawl in here. Real exercise makes me turn red and sweat. I can't do that. I wear a business suit all day." The picture he conjured up in my mind made me smile. I explained to him that

exercise done gradually didn't have to make him feel uncomfortable or get all red or even sweaty. A scientific exercise
program would progressively strengthen him physically, for-
tify him emotionally, and might even make him think more
clearly. The idea of being sharper appealed to Jack. He
wanted to be a leader who didn't look sick. After much discussion about what exercise would not be, Jack agreed to
start the program. In the following weeks of working with
him, Jack confided in me that as an adolescent boy he was
awkward and didn't run fast or see well enough to hit or
catch a ball. The taunting of his schoolmates had left an emotional scar and made him self-conscious. He was the laugh-
ingstock of the schoolyard, and the memories still bothered
him even though he had become extremely successful. "This
type of exercise," he said, "was different. It makes me feel better, stronger and more confident, but it also progresses so
gradually I can actually succeed in the program." Jack was
clearly proud of his accomplishments and has continued to
exercise long after his treatments ended.

EXERCISE PROGRAMS USED IN RESEARCH

A variety of exercise programs have been studied with cancer
patients. Some expect patients to exercise every day; others
require patients to exercise only three or four days a week.
Studies have looked at the benefits of exercise when patients
are allowed to exercise at home, in small groups, and in individual supervised exercise programs (one on one with a personal trainer). The type of exercise varies by study, too. Some
studies have allowed patients to choose an aerobic activity that
they enjoy, such as walking, cycling, or swimming; others have

dictated the activity, such as treadmill walking or running or riding a stationary bicycle. I think the best activities are those that keep you using the muscles we use in everyday life. I consider walking the best and safest activity because it is an activity we do everyday and is generally pretty easy to do in a neighborhood, on the local high school track, or in a shopping mall. Conveniently, walking does not require any expensive equipment besides a good pair of shoes. If walking is difficult because of physical problems or you simply need a little variety in your routine, other activities you might want to do include swimming, rowing, or stationary cycling. If you are confined to a bed, a bed bicycle is a terrific way to keep your legs strong enough that you can walk out of the hospital and your heart and lungs fit enough to keep you moving. If you are unable to use your legs, an arm cycle or rowing machine can help you maintain your strength and stamina. Regardless of the exercise prescription or setting, all of the studies of cancer patients receiving treatment either in the hospital or as outpatients report positive findings, and none have reported any adverse health problems for the participants.

EXERCISE FOR HOSPITALIZED PATIENTS

You probably don't think of exercise as part of a hospital regimen for cancer patients, and neither do most hospitals. The interest and the effort of determined physical therapists, nurses, exercise scientists, and some physicians is growing, however, and programs are being developed to keep patients active and strong during hospitalization to prevent some of the debilitating effects of inactivity and bed rest. Some cancer centers have gentle stretching and yoga programs, which don't do a lot for preventing the debilitating loss of muscle strength and cardiovascular endurance but can certainly help to keep muscles limber and may make patients feel better and more relaxed. A few cancer centers urge patients to walk the halls or even have a room with exercise equipment or exercise videos to follow. None of these programs are supervised or provide much in the way of guidelines for exercise, but interest is growing and health care providers are making efforts not only to cure their patients of cancer, but to keep them functioning during treatment and long into survivorship.

Research studies for the most part have focused on patients receiving outpatient treatments. However, a research team in Germany has developed an exercise program using a bed bicycle for patients receiving bone marrow transplants who are confined to the hospital for long periods of time, and it is one of my favorite programs. The bed bicycle program is performed every day in an effort to keep patients strong or to make them stronger to prevent some of the profound weakness and overwhelming fatigue experienced during hospitalization and following discharge. Patients simply lie in bed and pedal for a minute and then rest for a minute. The intensity of the exercise is in the range of 10 to 12 on the RPE chart. Lying in bed and pedaling is an easy form of exercise that is very achievable for the majority of cancer patients. I consider it the all-American exercise program; no other exercise program allows us to exercise while lying in bed playing video games, answering email, or filing our nails. If you cannot pedal with your legs, there are devices that allow you to pedal or row with your arms to keep them strong and, more important, to keep your heart and lungs from becoming too debilitated.

The vast majority of exercise programs used in research programs have focused on aerobic exercises, activities that are sustained, like walking. Some of my studies have looked at the effects of resistance exercises, like lifting weights or using resistance bands, on physical and emotional function. While resistance exercises certainly make folks stronger, people don't seem to enjoy them as much, and after several months many seem to prefer walking or another aerobic form of exercise. Following a resistance exercise program may require more determination and discipline to stick with the routine over time. However, resistance exercise is a terrific way to build or maintain your strength while in the hospital or confined to a bed or lounge chair. Undoubtedly the optimal program for health and fitness is a combination of aerobic and resistance exercises, which I will explain in later chapters.

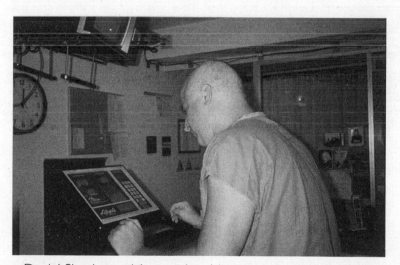

Daniel Shapiro pedals away in a bone marrow transplant unit

My studies of muscle strength have used Thera-Bands, which are somewhat like giant rubber bands. Thera-Bands are color coded, each color being a different degree of thickness, which creates more or less resistance. There are many ways to anchor the band so that you can pull on it; over a door, around the leg of a couch, standing on one end, or even securing it to part of a hospital bed. Depending on how you anchor the Thera-Band, you can strengthen most of the major muscles in your body. I will show you some pictures of these exercises in Chapters 8 and 9. Most hospitals do not offer physical rehabilitation programs for cancer patients, although you are given information as to the importance of exercise during cancer treatment. If there is no exercise area provided for you, advocate for yourself and other patients and ask for a bed bicycle or stationary bicycle or for some Thera-Bands to be brought into your room or even sent home with you.

REGAINING AND RETAINING YOUTHFULNESS

Ruby was 82 years young when I met her. She was working as a volunteer in the hospital gift shop and helping people find their way through the hospital halls. She was 80 years old when she was diagnosed with breast cancer and 81 years old when she completed all her treatments. When we met, she complained of a lack of stamina and was concerned about doing too much because her doctors had told her to "take it easy." She said, "All my life I've been a doer for myself, my family, and others. I can't just sit around, but now I'm afraid to go back to my old exercise routine that I've done for probably twenty years." Ruby's exercise program before her diagnosis consisted of walking 2 miles 3 days a week and water aerobics classes 2 to 3 days a week, in addition to her volunteer activities at the hospital and at a museum 3 days a week. She was a busy woman and devastated by her doctor's advice to take it easy and slow down. She proclaimed, "By following his advice I am getting old, but I'm afraid it might not be safe to exercise now." Ruby and I met only a few times. She simply needed a little reassurance that she could exercise safely. The hardest part of starting to exercise again for Ruby was learning to pace herself. She wanted to charge off at top speed and after a few minutes would get breathless and frustrated. "I used to walk like this every day; what's wrong with me?" Teaching her to be patient and let her body get strong and fit again was our biggest challenge. After several months of progressive and consistent exercise, she's back to her usual walking and water aerobics routine and feeling like she's getting younger.

Ruby's experience is very common for people of all ages. What we forget is that exercise and movement are critical for life. Our bodies are designed to move and be used. If we don't use our muscles and bodies, they don't work as well after a while. Ruby started a combined walking and resistance exercise program and after about 4 weeks declared that she was feeling much stronger and was getting through the day with more energy and spunk. What changed for her? She began to rebuild her muscle strength and her cardiovascular fitness.

INDIVIDUALIZING AN EXERCISE PROGRAM

Developing an exercise program, whether you are a "healthy" cancer patient or one who has become significantly debilitated from treatment or the effects of your disease, requires looking at you as an individual and creating a program designed specifically for you. The program needs to consider your current physical ability, physical limitations, past experience with exercise, and treatment regimen. Custom tailoring a program to your ability and physical needs involves considering such factors as the type and stage of cancer you have; the type of treatment(s) you are receiving or received; whether you are at risk of developing lymphedema (swelling of an arm or leg from surgery); if you have numbness in your feet or hands (peripheral neuropathy) as a result of some chemotherapies; and whether you have other chronic illnesses, such as arthritis, hypertension, or osteoporosis. These and many other conditions do not prevent you from exercising, but they may require some creativity in developing an exercise program that is safe and effective and, of course, makes you feel better and have fun.

Exercise is an ageless intervention if it is tailored to your abilities. Research studies are showing us the importance of exercise for people of all ages, shapes, and sizes in reducing risks for cancer recurrence and the development of secondary cancers and improving muscle strength and bone health while also reducing risks for osteoporosis, heart disease, diabetes, hypertension, and obesity. The following chapters will help you start one of the Cancer Fitness programs or build your own scientific and sensible aerobic or resistance exercise program that takes into account your fitness level and past experience with exercise. Adapting an exercise program to one's individual ability and physical limitations allows everyone to reap the benefits of exercise, get the most out of life, feel healthy, and improve their chances of long-term survival.

RUTH'S STORY

Ruth was 86 years old and living in a retirement center. When I met Ruth she had just been diagnosed with an early-stage breast cancer that required surgery but no further treatment. Her daughter confided in me that her mom was no longer able to get up out of the chair and was just not motivated to do anything for herself and demanding that people help her with everything. Other than being ornery and depressed about her cancer and living situation, she had her mind and was healthy and able, although not willing, to take care of herself. To help her out of the doldrums, we coordinated a Lawrence Welk sing-along and eventually created a dance-along program for her and invited the other residents of the facility. Although many of the residents danced while sitting in their chairs, some leaned on their walkers or chairs for support and moved with the music and others actually did a little jig in place. Ruth and the other residents enjoyed this movement and dance so much that it became a regular activity and was often spontaneously started at impromptu times when a resident would play some good old-time music. Over time, Ruth became more independent and started taking care of herself again and now gets snappy if her family tries to do too much for her, saying, with a twinkle in her eyes, "I can do that myself. Do you think I'm too old?"

KEY POINTS

- Exercise is safe for cancer patients.
- Exercise should be fun; not make you feel uncomfortable.

- Exercise programs should be individually tailored to your ability and needs.
- Use the rating of perceived exertion (RPE) scale to determine how hard you are exercising.
- Adapt exercise to match your physical abilities so you can reap the many physical and emotional rewards.

CHAPTER 6

CANCER FITNESS
AEROBIC EXERCISE PROGRAM

The aerobic exercise program in this chapter is the one that I use in my exercise studies and on which I start the vast majority of my patients. It is very simple and can be done in a 30-minute time period. If you are highly motivated and committed to doing a combined aerobic and resistance program, there are suggestions in Chapter 8 for combining the two programs . You may also want to combine the programs if your goal is to become stronger and increase your endurance, and you have some muscle weakness that you want to correct. Regardless of the program you choose, start slowly, progress consistently, and be patient. The guidelines for each of the programs will help you to start a scientifically tested and safe program. The information in Chapters 7 and 8 will help you learn how to modify the aerobic exercise programs to meet your specific goals and individual needs.

CHASING THREE CHILDREN

With stage III breast cancer and three children under the age of 4, Jody, age 39, was hardly able to keep up with her daily life. Her breast cancer treatment was aggressive, and the chemotherapy made her muscles ache. As her treatments progressed she didn't want to leave the house. Her friends would bring groceries and help with the children, and her husband did most of the chores around the house at night after work. Jody was spending more and more time on the couch, gaining weight and becoming increasingly weak. She no longer was able to walk from her favorite chair to her bedroom upstairs without becoming breathless and exhausted. The treatments and her physical changes caused great emotional anguish and despair. Even after her chemotherapy ended, she did not want to resume a more active lifestyle. Although she loved her children deeply and felt guilty for not being able to do more for them, she just didn't have the energy. With much coaxing Jody began walking; first to her mailbox and later around the small pond by her home. Eventually Jody joined a women's walking group of Cancer Fitness graduates. The group was terrifically supportive and encouraging. Her walking companions urged her to join them on a regular basis and would call her before their walks to be sure she would be going with them. The group support, the regular aerobic exercise, and the help of an antidepressant assisted Jody to return to a full life. It took great effort for her to commit to walking with the group 3 days a week, but she did and slowly began losing weight and feeling like her old self again. She told me, "If I hadn't started walking with my new friends, I don't know what would have happened to me. I was at the bottom and saw no way out. Even those short walks to the pond helped me to believe I might be able to get my life back."

CANCER FITNESS AEROBIC EXERCISE PROGRAM

To begin the Cancer Fitness aerobic exercise program, select an aerobic activity (e.g., walking, bicycling, swimming, or rowing) that you enjoy and will continue to do over time; for most people I suggest walking. To start, just complete the recommended exercise time and work at a rating of perceived exertion (RPE) between 11 and 14 (see Chapter 5). This means you will be exercising at a pace that makes you breath harder than if you were just moving around the house, but you can still carry on a conversation. As you build your endurance, start to push your pace, move a little faster, and aim to exercise at an RPE of 13 to 15—at a pace that makes you breath hard but steady and can still talk but have to concentrate a little more on talking between breaths. You don't have to start running, just walk or bicycle or do your favorite activity a little harder. If you live in a hilly place, push the pace for a minute or so as you go up a hill. If you are exercising in your living room or neighborhood gym on a treadmill, stair stepper, or other stationary equipment, turn up the speed for 15 or 20 seconds or increase the incline 1 or 2 percent for a short period of time to mimic going up a hill.

Does this program seem too much to start with? Cut the recommended time in half, or even more if you need to, and gradually work up to the starting point of the program. If you need to break the sessions into shorter periods of time you will still receive benefits. Science has shown us that mul-

Table 2. Cancer Fitness Aerobic Exercise Program

How often do I need to exercise aerobically? Exercise 3 to 4 days a week or every other day with a rest day between.

How hard or fast do I have to exercise aerobically? Exercise within your ability and comfort. The exercise should be at a pace to allow you to carry on a conversation. Intensity, how hard or fast you go, should be controlled by how you feel and any unusual symptoms you experience. If you feel uncomfortable, slow down. If you continue to feel bad, stop the exercise. Exercise at a RPE of 11 to 14 if you are on treatment and 13 to 15 if you are off treatment and starting to feel pretty strong.

How long do I have to exercise? This will depend on what week you are on. The exercise plan slowly increases the amount of exercise you do each week, peaking at a maximum of 30 minutes a day.

How does this work with chemotherapy weeks? The exercise program progresses pretty slowly and most of my patients do not have a problem keeping up with the progression, but if you are struggling with side effects from your treatment, then on your treatment weeks go back and do the exercise recommended for the two weeks before. Say, for example, you get treatment on week 1 and complete the exercise just fine but struggle with your side effects, you succeed in completing weeks 2 and 3, and at the beginning of week 4 you are going to get chemotherapy.

Instead of starting the week 4 exercise, go back and repeat week 2, and then the following weeks continue with week 3 and 4 until your next chemotherapy, when you will drop back and start with week 3.

Remember: In your exercise log (see Chapter 4), keep track of how long you exercise (number of minutes), how you felt, and your rating of perceived exertion (RPE).

How long to exercise? Remember, if you need to decrease the time or break the exercise up into several different exercise sessions, that's fine. Be patient and gradually work up to the recommended exercise times. Your body will get stronger, it just takes time.

Let's Get Going

Week 1:   Day 1: 15 minutes
            Day 2: 18 minutes
            Day 3: 20 minutes

Week 2:   Day 1: 18 minutes
            Day 2: 22 minutes
            Day 3: 25 minutes

Week 3:   Day 1: 20 minutes
            Day 2: 24 minutes
            Day 3: 27 minutes

Week 4:   Day 1: 23 minutes
            Day 2: 26 minutes
            Day 3: 30 minutes

Week 5:   Day 1: 20 minutes
            Day 2: 24 minutes
            Day 3: 27 minutes

Week 6:   Day 1: 23 minutes
            Day 2: 26 minutes
            Day 3: 30 minutes

Week 7:   Day 1: 20 minutes
            Day 2: 24 minutes
            Day 3: 27 minutes

Week 8:   Day 1: 23 minutes
            Day 2: 26 minutes
            Day 3: 30 minutes

Beyond Week 8 At this point you are now in an exercise routine. Go back to week 4 and start working forward again toward week 8. Try to increase your intensity—push yourself a little harder by increasing your RPE. You can keep your duration of exercise the same, or if you feel like it, gradually increase the amount of time that you exercise. What is important is that you keep exercising consistently. If you can fit it in your life, add a few more minutes of exercise to your program.

tiple sessions of exercise in a day accumulate and contribute to building your fitness. So, if you can only walk or exercise for 1 or 2 minutes and then need to rest, do that. Later in the day complete another 1 or 2 minutes of exercise. Gradually, over time, you will be able to exercise for a longer period of time and will be able to do more exercise in one session. Our bodies are amazing—a little physical activity and they start to get strong and fit once again. Those activities that you never thought you could do again become attainable, but not without a steady commitment to making exercise a part of your life.

COMING BACK TO LIFE

Angie was a proud, middle-aged woman with lung cancer who was emotionally overwhelmed by chemotherapy, being bald, and the changes in her appearance. She was so consumed by her physical changes that she had not left her house, except to go for treatment, in nearly 4 months. During this time she had gotten progressively weaker, debilitated, and depressed, to the point that she needed to use a wheelchair to get from the parking lot to her doctor's office. She was losing her will to live and saw absolutely no joy in life. I suggested that she begin increasing her physical activity by walking the distance of her living room at least once each day, any 4 days of the week she chose. The following week we increased her living room walking to 3 times a day, 4 or 5 days of the week. When she came back to clinic she proclaimed, "I didn't do what you told me to do last week." She paused waiting to see my reaction, and then, with a glimmer in her eye, said, "I started walking outside! I can nearly go all the way to the end of the block, and I walked in here from the parking lot!" For the first time in many months she was smiling and seemed to be sitting up a little straighter and feeling more confident. Her parting words were, "Exercise is the best medicine. I'm coming back to life!"

CHAPTER 7

ATHLETES:
CREATE YOUR OWN
EXERCISE PROGRAM

This chapter will help you develop the knowledge to create your own exercise program, modify the Cancer Fitness aerobic exercise program to your individual needs, and know when to take rest days or increase your exercise intensity. This chapter is for anyone interested in knowing how to exercise successfully in a scientific and efficient manner. The beginning exerciser may not be interested in all of the details but may find the information on how to handle sick days or overtraining useful, while the more serious exerciser may find the information about how to structure a training plan or peak for a specific event of particular interest. What I hope you will learn in this chapter is that more exercise is not better, but rather that the quality of your exercise is what makes the difference.

WHERE TO START?

Knowing how much exercise to do when you first start a program is difficult. I always recommend starting off doing much less than you think you can or should do. Not only do I want you to succeed at starting an exercise program, but also I don't want you to feel uncomfortable. Remember, if you are going to make exercise part of your life, you have a long time to get fit and you must slowly and steadily develop a routine that you enjoy.

If you were a regular exerciser before cancer and are currently receiving treatment or your treatment has ended and you want to regain your form, start slowly. I can't emphasize enough the importance of starting slowly. Trying to resume your previous exercise program isn't reasonable. Although you may succeed for a few days, the fitness loss will catch up with you. People usually experience remarkable fatigue and muscle soreness and show signs of becoming overtrained. I suggest cutting your usual activity in half and starting with a few easy days of cycling, swimming, or whatever your sport is. Listen to your body. You will get your fitness back, but it will take time and patience. Starting back with high-intensity training may set you up for failure by your not being able to complete your exercise plan for the day and by creating utter exhaustion. Train smart: develop a sensible exercise or training program, and keep a log of your progress and how you feel. The information in this chapter will help you to develop an exercise program based on different cycles of exercise, some more challenging than others, all gradually and systematically building on themselves.

Coming back after a prolonged period of inactivity and cancer treatment is not like starting to exercise for the first time. Everyone encounters highs and lows in performance and ability. The ups and downs during and following cancer treatment can be deeper and more unpredictable than recovery from other illnesses and may be related to treatment-related fatigue or other lingering side effects. For example, you may experience acute or long-lasting side effects of treatment that may slow you down and reduce your ability to tolerate intense activity. You may even experience new permanent physical changes that may limit your ability to exercise, such as numbness in your feet, which affects balance, walking, and nearly every activity we do on our feet, or a change in muscle balance because of surgery. With time, patience, and persistence, you will learn how to exercise and live a full life despite these limitations. However, I have had some patients who actually changed their activity because of the severe and lasting side effects of treatment.

OVERCOMING NEW PHYSICAL LIMITATIONS

Randy was 19 years old and an all-around athlete competing in high school track, swimming, and baseball. He had just received a college track scholarship when he was diagnosed with a sarcoma, a bony tumor, in his hamstring. Extensive surgery was required to remove the tumor and a large part of muscle, which was followed by chemotherapy and radiation therapy. Every day he worked diligently on stretching his leg and working out the fibrous adhesions on his scar, which ran from his buttocks to his knee. When he was in the hospital receiving chemotherapy, he worked on walking and being able to pull his knee up to his chest. By the end of chemotherapy, he was able to walk easily and had started riding a stationary bicycle. In the first several weeks of cycling he was able to pedal only a minute or two and then needed to rest, but by the end of chemotherapy, nearly 4 months later, he could pedal 20 minutes in one continuous stretch. Although Randy would be able to function normally in daily life, he learned that his hamstring strength would never be what it was because the surgery had disrupted one of his hamstring muscles. This meant that Randy wouldn't be able to be the top-notch sprinter he was before diagnosis. After many months of struggling with this reality and working with weights to get his strength back, he came to understand that if he wanted to compete he needed to choose another sport. Randy started swimming, and after 6 months of continuous training he was swimming faster than he did in high school and aiming to compete in college on a swimming scholarship.

WHY ARE YOU EXERCISING?

You need to ask yourself why you are exercising. To reduce fatigue? Lose weight? Maintain or increase your strength? If managing your fatigue and some of the other side effects associated with treatment is your primary reason for exercising, following the Cancer Fitness aerobic exercise program will help you and may be simpler than creating your own exercise program. However, if you have completed treatment and your primary goal is to shed some excess weight that accumulated during your cancer treatment or over the course of aging, then you may want to take a different approach. Begin by following the Cancer Fitness aerobic exercise program for 8 weeks. After an 8-week period of consistent exercise, you should feel strong enough to begin to increase your duration, or time, of exercise without feeling completely exhausted. To facilitate weight loss it will be important for you to exercise 30 to 45 minutes 3 or 4 days a week, and make modifications to your diet—reduce calorie and fat intake and increase fruits, vegetables, and low-fat foods. You may also want to add resistance exercise to your regimen. Resistance exercise helps to build your muscles, and, conveniently, stronger muscles burn more calories. If weight loss is your goal, try to exercise 4 or 5 days a week

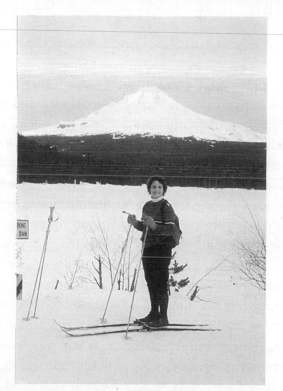

"Never too old for a great day of exercise." Janet Smith goes cross-country skiing at Trillium Lake near Mt. Hood, Oregon.

with two of the exercise sessions at a moderate intensity (RPE 13 to 15) and longer duration, one exercise session at a lower intensity (RPE 11 to 13) and longer duration, and the other at a higher intensity (RPE 14 to 16) but for a shorter duration. If you were to add resistance exercise to your regimen, do your aerobic exercise first and then the resistance exercise. This will allow your muscles to get a good warm-up and make it so that your muscles aren't too tired from the resistance exercise to perform during your aerobic workout, or you may complete the resistance exercises on a different day.

MAKING YOUR OWN EXERCISE PLAN

Everyone needs an exercise plan, regardless of your level of physical activity or your goal. A plan makes it easier to go out and follow through with your activity, gives you a goal to attain, gives a focus to your exercise routine, and helps prevent boredom. Your exercise plan needs to be detailed, with reasonable and attainable goals for each exercise session. Your plan should be directed toward maintaining a regular exercise program or specific enough to take you up to the day of a particular event. The plan will be divided into cycles, each focusing on specific activities and amounts of exercise. The three cycles are *microcycle, mesocycle,* and *macrocycle.*

A *microcycle* is the duration of a week and is equivalent to one week of exercise (Table 3). Microcycles are designed to include specificity in each workout. If you have competitive goals in mind or simply want to push yourself to become stronger and faster, each exercise session will need to focus on developing a different aspect of your physiology. Some days you will go at a steady aerobic pace, some days you will

Table 3. Example of a Microcycle for a Walker

Monday: Rest day or active recovery. If active recovery, a leisurely walk for 15 minutes at an RPE of 10 to 11.

Tuesday: Anaerobic work or speed work. Warm up at a leisurely pace for 5 minutes and then walk at top speed for 10 seconds. Recover at a slow walk and repeat 3 times. Take as much time as you need to recover. When you get stronger, 20 to 30 seconds should be enough. Cool down by walking at a leisurely speed for 5 minutes. Your RPE for the fast walk should be between 13 and 15.

Wednesday: Endurance walk at a steady pace for 20 to 30 minutes. Walk at an RPE of 12.

Thursday: 20 to 30 minutes. After you warm up for 5 to 10 minutes, walk at a brisk pace for 2 minutes. Slow down and recover for 2 minutes, and then walk briskly for another 2 minutes. Repeat this sequence one more time. Do the 2-minute efforts at an RPE of 14 to 15. Recover at an RPE of 9 or 10. Cool down before you quit.

Friday: Rest day or active recovery (see Monday).

Saturday and/or Sunday: Walk with group, pushing the pace up short hills, going easy on the downhill. Keep your RPE between 11 and 14.

periodically increase your intensity to an anaerobic pace, and other days you will focus on longer bursts of speed at a moderate, or submaximal, intensity. By stressing the different metabolic pathways in our bodies, we become fitter and faster. Rest days are some of the most difficult days to follow; it requires remarkable self-discipline to go at an easy pace, not the usual pace of most of your exercise days. I know some of you will find this hard to believe, but once you start this program you will see that it is easiest to go at a medium speed for every workout. Varying your pace from higher intensity to very low intensity is more challenging than one might expect. Most people find that going supereasy on a recovery day takes a lot of willpower and awareness of your breathing and heart rate. These easy rest and recovery days are the secret to many top performances in sport.

Table 3 may scare you into thinking you have to exercise every day. You don't! You can take rest days as days off and aim to exercise three days a week, or exercise every other day. What's important is that you get out there and exercise, not which day of the week you do it. There's no magic in the days, but you will need a day off between some of your workouts. I find that varying your workout, so that some days you push yourself and other days you go easy, helps to reduce monotony, and science has certainly demonstrated that rest days are essential to realize gains in your fitness. A structured exercise program or routine is not only what I recommend for my patients, but it is the way athletes train whether they are planning for a 100-meter sprint or a marathon.

A *mesocycle* is a period of time lasting about one month or the equivalent of three or four microcycles (Table 4). The length of a mesocycle is determined in part by your level of fitness. If you are just beginning an exercise program, have been very ill, or are just starting back to exercise, don't over-

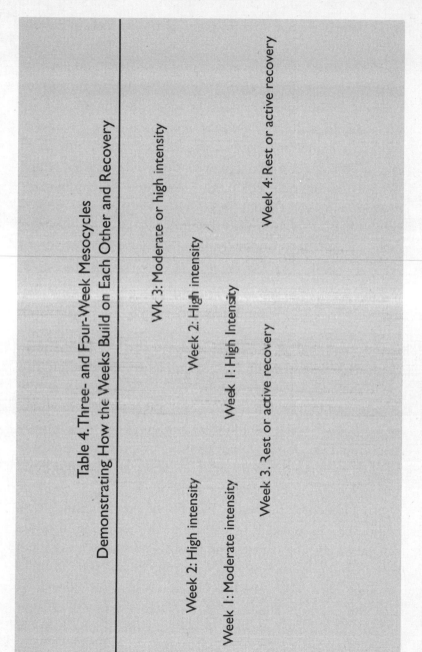

Table 4. Three- and Four-Week Mesocycles
Demonstrating How the Weeks Build on Each Other and Recovery

Week 1: Moderate intensity

Week 2: High intensity

Wk 3: Moderate or high intensity

Week 1: High Intensity

Week 2: High intensity

Week 3. Rest or active recovery

Week 4: Rest or active recovery

stress your body. Set up a program of three weeks per cycle so that you get adequate recovery time between each step up in the program. When your body is stronger and you can tolerate more exercise, then you will be able to move successfully to four-week cycles. The weeks in a mesocycle are broken into different intensity levels, from easy recovery weeks to higher intensity workouts, or what I call "hard weeks." If you choose to start with three-week cycles, which is what I recommend for anyone starting a structured exercise program, you should begin with two weeks of moderate- to hard-intensity exercise and then take a week of rest, or you could begin with two moderate weeks followed by a recovery week. The rest or easy recovery week consists of reducing the duration of your activity and the intensity, which means spending less time exercising and exercising at a lower level, or RPE, that does not push you physically. This is the week that your body recuperates to be able to push you to a new level. Sound appealing? The hard weeks in this cycle includes some speed work (very short high-intensity efforts) and longer durations of exercise at a lower intensity, or RPE. Each week the intensity and duration of your exercise should vary. Varying your exercise program will not only help to train the different physiologic systems in your body but will help prevent staleness and boredom.

In addition to the fitness benefits of exercising in cycles, mesocycles have health benefits, too. By exercising in cycles you avoid pushing yourself too hard and reduce your chances of becoming injured or sick. This type of scientific exercise program also helps your body accommodate to exercise so that you can enjoy the benefits of reducing your risk of heart disease, high blood pressure, diabetes, arthritis, and burning more calories, which helps with weight control.

Table 5. Macrocycle Pattern Showing How One Week Builds on Another and Then an Easy Week Cuts Down the Intensity and Workload

Easy

Moderate

Moderate   Easy

Moderate   Moderate   Easy

Hard   Moderate   Moderate   Easy

Hard   Moderate   Moderate   Easy

Hard   Moderate   Easy

Hard   Moderate

Moderate

The long-term overview of your exercise plan is called a *macrocycle*. Table 5 illustrates how weeks of varying intensity build into mesocycles, which then become macrocycles. Macrocycles can range from several months to years and reflect, if you keep a log and can track your exercise, all the exercise that you do over a period of months and years.

MORE ON EXERCISE LOGS

It is important to keep an exercise log that includes what you had planned to do, what you really did, and how you felt. Over the period of several mesocycles, you will begin to learn your body's patterns of adapting to exercise and see how the weather influenced your workout or how a micro- or mesocycle may have caused too much fatigue or even led to an injury. The best part of an exercise log is that it is motivating. You can easily chart your progress and see how you are able to tolerate more intensity, harder workouts, and longer workouts, whether that means walking one lap around the hospital ward or running around the local park. I often feel as though I'm not getting anywhere with my exercise program, but when I look back at my log I can see that I steadily go farther and don't get as tired as I did a few weeks ago.

TAPERING

There are always days when you want to be in top form and have a truly stellar performance, even if you aren't training for a specific event. This top performance goal could be setting the pace and leading the walking group on your long walk. You can make this peak performance happen by tapering. *Tapering* is cutting back on your activity so that you are in optimal condition at a certain time. The taper is often the hardest part of the plan. It takes discipline to let your body recover fully. During this time, it is vital to optimize your rest and nutrition, decrease stress, and spend time visualizing how you will look, feel, and push through to your top performance during your event. If you are tapering for a one-day event, the taper week will include some specificity a day or two before the event. The two to three days before the event should be easy, active recovery days: get out and move around, but don't push yourself to set a personal best. Hold back until the day you want to have the best performance. While you are in your recovery taper phase, you should be focusing your thoughts on your big day, not on what you should have done to be faster or have more endurance. It's too late for that; you've done what you've done, and heavy training now will not make up for poor training in the previous weeks. The taper period is a good time to examine how you feel (rested, tight, confident, or anxious) and focus your energies on resting, stretching, and visualizing.

> When I had a plan to follow and gently and steadily got in shape, I felt better and had more confidence and self-esteem. Transforming from a nonexerciser to a regular exerciser made a difference in how I looked, felt, and was able to handle life's challenges.
>
> —Janice, 51 years old, with lung cancer

QUALITY VERSUS QUANTITY

More repetitions or longer durations of exercise are not necessarily better. It is far more important to do the exercise correctly and at the proper intensity or RPE. If you are seeking higher levels of fitness, have successfully completed the Cancer Fitness aerobic exercise program, and are building intervals (periods of higher intensity exercise that can last from a few seconds to several minutes) into your exercise training plan, you will be ready to work at higher intensity levels. Don't aim for doing 8 or 12 aerobic intervals because it sounds like a lot and more must make you fitter and faster. Do 3 or 4 aerobic intervals at 100 percent effort.

In all my years of coaching cyclists, one of my biggest joys was teaching people to really give 100 percent effort. I consistently worked with athletes who insisted that they were going 100 percent and couldn't possibly go any harder. Through specific drills I would teach them they could give a whole lot more. Each time they finished an effort I asked them to tell me how hard they went. Some of them took eight or ten tries to really figure out that their previous efforts at "100 percent" were really only about 75 percent of their best effort. When these athletes learned to give 100 or 110 percent, they were amazed at how they performed. They quickly learned that quality efforts are key to going fast and getting stronger. Short, hard efforts produce faster results than mediocre efforts, which don't do much except make you tired because you spend too much time working out in a no-man's-land. That's why I tell you in the Cancer Fitness aerobic exercise program that when you can exercise continuously for 30 minutes, cut back your duration of exercise and increase your pace or intensity. Of course there are exceptions: if your goal is to ride a century (100 miles) or run a marathon you will need to exercise for longer periods of time. Whether you exercise for 30 minutes or several hours, I know that if you use these training techniques you will see rapid results and be able to have a life outside of your exercise program, too, because you'll spend less time exercising!

A TIME FOR EVERYTHING

Early in my cycling career I decided to ride in an event called Bicycle Across Missouri (BAM). The event covers 587 long, hilly miles, and official finishers must complete the ride in 63 hours or less. I had carefully calculated my riding times and planned to send food ahead to each of the checkpoints. Based on my previous long rides, I had calculated my speed and arrival time at each checkpoint where I might need spare batteries or a warmer jersey and tights for the night. The plan was precise, and I had a large seat pack to carry lights, snacks, rain jacket, and equipment to change a flat. I did what I thought was adequate training in the "hills" of northern Florida and then flew to St. Louis where, on the way to the hotel, I saw real hills—steep, long ones! I was overwhelmed by the sight, checked in, and immediately decided a nap would make the hills look better. Two hours later, I looked out the window of my room. The hills were still there and just as big, but now a lot of activity was going on in the parking lot. I decided to go and check out the fun.

Big rigs, motor homes for the riders to rest in, follow vehicles with enormous light racks mounted on the rooftop, riders with two and three bicycles, every rider with at least one crew person to support them on their ride.

What was I doing? When I registered and collected my number, the boys at the registration table laughed and said they were waiting to meet the gal from Florida going unsupported. "Not many men complete this ride unsupported unless they hook up with another crew," they advised. I told them I was sure that wouldn't be a problem. If my eyes didn't give me away I would be surprised. I knew I was in for an adventure!

At 6 A.M. we gather at the start. Kindly folks tell me to ride at my own pace, that the first 100 miles are the toughest, with unrelenting hills. Okay, I'll pace myself. We start and I ride with a group of men in their 50s. I'm hanging with them and starting to feel like this may not be such a bad experience, until we meet Highway T, which stands for Terrible Hills. The first climb I go 110 percent and barely hang with the men; climbs 2 and 3 I get "gently" dropped but reconnect with them on the descent. Then I'm on my own alone in a sea of endless hills that swallow me up at the bottom as I struggle to keep some momentum to pedal up the other side. The first rest stop is at 25 miles. I decide it's too early to stop; besides, I'm way off my time schedule. So, I push on and do not get the drinks and food I had stashed there. I begin to realize that weight is the enemy, and I am carrying lots of extra weight on my very own body! As I talk to myself about dieting and losing weight I determine that I will start today. Why not start today? No excuses or reasons to procrastinate. The 50-mile rest stop—stretch, get some water, and pedal on. I can see that I am losing time and don't see any way to get back on my schedule, which means that I won't arrive by nightfall to the checkpoint where I have sent my night-riding clothes. Even through the roads are very quiet, I am still afraid of not being visible in the dark, so I start to push myself to ride faster. At the 100-mile rest stop I eat one PowerBar. It seems like it should be enough; after all, I am on a diet and will be sleek and trim by the end of the event. (Had I already lost common sense? I knew better than this, but the illogical voices were clearly winning out.)

Nightfall came and I had a small front and rear light. Not much light for rural Missouri roads, but enough to get by. I only rode off the road once, and then it was into a freshly plowed cornfield. After riding a little over 21 hours at an average of 13 miles an hour, I arrived at the halfway point exhausted and downhearted. It was after 2 A.M., I had ridden further than I had ever gone before, but I was supposed to be here 2 hours earlier! How could I have miscalculated? How could I possibly be riding so slowly? I refused to let the idea that I hadn't been eating or drinking factor into my performance. I wasn't thinking clearly either, as I decided that there was no conceivable way that I could complete the ride within the official time. So, I decided to drop out. With that decision made, it then occurred to me that I was stuck in Kansas City with no way back to St. Louis! I started offering myself as crew in exchange for a ride back to St. Louis for my bike and me. Eventually, I met another rider whose wife was the only crew member and who was delighted to have me for company and help. As I sat and rested I felt the terrible feelings of failure and then the grim realization that I quit far too soon. I had completely miscalculated and given up too quickly. Twenty-one plus twenty-one was not eighty something. I would easily have finished within the 63-hour time limit. As I got warm and ate a little food, I started to feel better physically and realized how silly and downright stupid my diet idea had been. Not only did it make me feel terrible, but I couldn't think.

BAM was a lesson in learning to pace myself, be reasonable in my decisions and expectations, and learn the importance of nutrition and hydration. Our bodies have to be properly fueled, even if we are carrying an extra 30 or 50 pounds that we don't like. There's a time for dieting, training, and pacing, and we all have to learn to set reasonable goals and push beyond our limits. I can laugh at myself, and I hope you will too as you use my foolishness to avoid your own mistakes.

OVERTRAINING

Human personalities differ widely. Some may want to exercise to excess, while others may not want to move at all. As you begin or resume your exercise program, take the time to find the right balance between pushing yourself too hard and not pushing yourself enough. Training in the cycles just described can help prevent injury as well as excessive overload on your muscles and cardiovascular system. Nearly every person I have coached has wanted to push to excess, resulting in overtraining, which usually causes fatigue, insomnia, irritability, and poor performance. No matter how hard you push yourself, your body just can't do what it could before. It's remarkably frustrating. If you're stubborn and continue to try to exercise beyond your current ability, you not only worsen the fatigue and overtraining syndrome so that it takes longer to recover, you also put yourself at increased risk of injury and of getting a viral infection, such as an upper respiratory infection. Overtraining counteracts the benefits of exercise during and following cancer treatment.

Overtraining doesn't go away by trying harder or working out longer; rest is the key to scratching your way out of the downward spiral. The sooner you recognize that you have been pushing yourself for too long, the sooner you can get back on your exercise training schedule, but only after several days of active recovery or real rest (no activity). For aggressive type A personalities, it may be hard to hold back, take rest days, and listen to your body. For the less driven and intense exerciser, the idea of overtraining may seem nearly impossible, but if you become committed to starting an exercise program, even if you aren't seeking to be competitive, you can become overtrained.

> Learning to pace myself and judge how easy to go on rest days was the hardest part of my exercise program. At first I kept pushing, even on rest days, and then I got frustrated because I couldn't run as fast or as far. I felt tired all the time and I wasn't sleeping well. The harder I pushed the worse I performed. After several days of fighting myself, I wondered if I was experiencing being overtrained? I took three days off with no activity and then started back to running short easy distances. Boy, did I feel better, but those three days of no exercise were hard!
>
> —Larry, a 63-year-old business executive
> with leukemia

MISSED EXERCISE DAYS:
WEATHER, ILLNESS, AND THE UNEXPECTED

Of course there will be times when because of illness, weather, and other unforeseen circumstances, you must change your exercise plan. This is expected, and even cheered by some. If you have to miss a few days of exercise because of foul weather, simply pick up your exercise program on the workout you had planned for today. Don't go back and try to pick things up or make up missed exercise sessions, just move forward from today's date. On the other hand, if illness forces you to miss a few days or a week of exercise, don't start back on whatever the plan was for today. Instead, start off with 2 or 3 very easy or light days of exercise. Listen to your body, and let your breathing, muscles and energy level guide you toward resuming your exercise plan.

Sam's story illustrates how important modifying your exercise program is to being able to exercise during treatment. Sam was a 34-year-old competitive marathon runner when he was diagnosed with stage III melanoma. His treatment included surgery, followed by high doses of interferon-alpha nearly every day for a year. Interferon-alpha is a drug that causes flulike side effects and profound fatigue and often causes people to stop working and not be able to do much more than lie on the couch. It is one of the most unpleasant immunotherapy drugs used. Fatigue can be so severe from interferon-alpha that the dose of the medication is often reduced. Sam dreaded the idea of treatment and losing his fitness, but the alternative, possible death from his disease, was even bleaker. So with great trepidation and reluctance he started the treatment and at the same time enrolled in one of my exercise programs. I asked Sam to limit his exercise to 4 days a week and to exercise at half his usual intensity. Sam was driven and didn't want to lose his fitness, but with a little coaxing and a systematic review of this running program, Sam eventually agreed to cut his exercise program in half. He religiously exercised 4 days a week. After the first 6 weeks of interferon-alpha treatment he told me, "There was no way I could have maintained my usual routine. If I hadn't followed your advice I would have pushed so hard that I couldn't keep exercising, and probably would have stopped my routine entirely."

Although Sam was not able to train at his usual intensity, the modified running program allowed him to continue running throughout his treatment. Sam told me that running helped him to combat his fatigue and depression and kept his energy at a level at which he could do most of his usual activities. Near the end of his treatment he told me, "my training has never been this light but I don't think I could have done any more. Four days of exercise was enough to make me feel better emotionally and still stay in reasonable condition physically."

PEAK PERFORMANCE

What is peaking? *Peaking* is being in your best form, having the best performance on the day that you need it to count. Being in optimal physical and psychological condition for a major event, such as a being the walk leader, running a race, going to an interview, or taking a test. How do you do it? These are questions to which no one has a definite answer. Peaking at just the right time is both an art and a science. If athletes and coaches knew more about how to peak, more records would be broken. Correct training and careful attention to your body will help you reach your maximum performance at the right time. Your program needs to be structured with specific times of more intense effort and time for rest and recovery. If you are training for a specific event, such as climbing a mountain, a bicycle trip, or a 5K race, you will want to do that specific activity (e.g., hiking, bicycling, walking, or running) and develop your exercise program to build on periodization. *Periodization* is the organized structure of training over an extended period of time in cycles (microcycle, mesocycle, and macrocycle).

Performing to the best of your potential at every exercise session or planned event would be optimal but is certainly not possible. If you have a group walk or bicycle ride every weekend, you will have natural days of feeling really strong and as though you could go forever and days when you just can't seem to hit your stride. Some of these ups and downs are related to the rigors of life, health, stress, work, and your exercise program. Assuming you are a weekend warrior and meet a group for a run or a bicycle ride every weekend, it is not reasonable to taper before each weekend. This approach would leave you in poor condition! I suggest choosing a few (one to three) events for which you would like to peak. Be sure the events are spaced by at least six weeks so that your body and mind have time to rest, recover, and refocus before the next training cycle and maximum effort. Some events that my patients have trained to peak for include (1) playing with grandchildren who will be visiting in two months; (2) keeping up with the walking, running, or cycling group;

(3) participating in the Danskin Triathlon; (3) climbing Mount Rainier; (4) cycling across the United States; (5) backpacking in the Grand Canyon, or (6) training to compete or win a national championship. To reach these goals, each of these athletes had to make a structured, progressive exercise plan to keep them focused on reaching their goal and to build in the time before their event to rest and recover, enabling them to have a peak performance.

PEAKING ON DEMAND

How do you set up your training program to peak on demand? Get a calendar and mark the events for which you plan to peak. Now, count back the number of weeks from the day of the event to the present date. Evaluate your fitness and exercise tolerance. Are three- or four-week cycles (mesocycles) best for you? Be realistic. You want to avoid pushing yourself too hard and becoming overtrained. Now, count the mesocycles from the present date to the day of the event. Depending on the length of the event for which you are peaking, you will need to build in a taper or active recovery period for at least one week before your big day. Now, plan your weeks to include hard, moderate, and recovery weeks. Do this up to the day of the event. Remember, the last week of your plan must be active recovery!

Before many big events, weekend warriors and elite athletes alike often feel incredibly exhausted. Our bodies pull in and begin to conserve energy. This fatigue phenomenon is normal; when your big day comes, you will feel invigorated and ready to reach your maximum potential.

In 1990 I set my first 24-hour distance cycling record, riding 418 miles around a 15-mile square in southern Florida. In the two-week recovery taper period before the event I felt overwhelmingly fatigued. My legs were heavy and tired and I just felt glued to the bed. All I wanted to do was sleep. I had never experienced this feeling before and couldn't imagine how in the past weeks I had ridden hundreds of miles. I couldn't even imagine riding 12 miles. I was experiencing anticipatory stress. My body was withdrawing and collecting its energies for the biggest competitive event of my life. The night before the event I had a forboding feeling and I still felt that riding a bike was a dream. I wondered what had gotten into me to think I could do this, and why had I told so many people, and even informed the media (oh no!) that I was going to attempt to break a record that had stood for over 10 years? Was I nuts? Fortunately, the next morning I woke up feeling alive and full of energy again. My legs felt rested and ready to work, and I was completely focused on sustaining my target heart rate, maintaining an aerodynamic position, and staying on pace. Now I notice that every time I have tried to peak for an event, whether it was another world record or an extended hiking trip in the Grand Canyon, I get that same incredible feeling of fatigue. It is the way my body works to recover actively and prepare. You will learn how your body responds to recovery and stress. Don't despair: you too will rise to the occasion and perform to your best ability.

SUMMARY

This chapter has reviewed the scientific basis of developing a safe and effective exercise plan. You can use this information to modify the Cancer Fitness aerobic exercise program or to develop your own program. Developing a training program tailored to your ability and realistic personal goals will help you to reach your goals and assure that you achieve your peak performance at the desired time. The most important part of exercise is learning to listen to your body and interpret what it tells you. Are you tired because of emotion or because you are physically pushing yourself too hard? Your body's messages are a critical component to developing fitness, avoiding overtraining, knowing when to start exercising after an illness, and achieving your personal goals and your peak performance.

CHAPTER 8

THE CORE OF RESISTANCE EXERCISE

This chapter provides information on the basics of resistance exercise and the structured detail necessary for those of you who want to develop your own resistance exercise program beyond the Cancer Fitness resistance exercise program, perhaps with the intention of focusing more on body sculpting or muscle building. Like the previous chapter, this chapter will develop your knowledge to create a scientifically sound, effective, and safe program.

MUSCLE ADAPTATION
TO RESISTANCE EXERCISE

Our muscle strength and muscle endurance are increased through work or overload. Muscles adapt to the demands of exercise and gradually become stronger and better able to withstand the stresses of everyday activity and exercise. Overloading the muscles is most commonly achieved through *resistance exercise,* or weight training. The muscle responds to the overload of resistance exercise by increasing the size of the muscle fiber and increasing the lean muscle mass in the body. Resistance exercises not only strengthen and improve muscle endurance but also improve the muscle's ability to recover from different forces and activities. Because you get stronger with resistance exercise, it becomes easier to perform your daily activities, and as in aerobic exercise you will feel a greater sense of self-confidence and possibly even self-worth. Another benefit of resistance exercise is that the increased lean muscle in your body burns more calories than fat does, which means that even when you are resting you will burn more calories per day than when you had less muscle mass before you started to follow a resistance exercise program.

Research has also shown that resistance training can reduce body fat, glucose tolerance, and blood lipid levels and improve bone density. All this means that resistance exercise can reduce your risks for heart disease, adult-onset diabetes, and osteoporosis. Resistance exercise strengthens not just your muscles but also the connective tissue around your joints and your bones. Strong muscles and connective tissues mean that you can recruit more muscular force and power to prevent or at least reduce your risk of injury from falls, muscle strains, and sprains. Resistance exercise puts strain on your bones, which, very simply stated, stimulates the bone to build more bone and increases bone density and mass, ultimately reducing your risks for osteoporosis. There is even research suggesting that regular resistance exercises may slow the natural deterioration and degeneration of aging. These studies have shown that people who are sedentary lose about 20 to 30 percent of their muscle mass by age 65. In contrast, those people in the study who performed resistance exercise maintained and even gained muscle.

REDUCING HEALTH RISKS

Bob and Ruth were a distinguished, sedentary elderly couple who both preferred reading a good book and eating a splendidly rich French meal to almost anything in life. At age 78, Bob was diagnosed with prostate cancer and began a treatment regimen that caused his muscles to atrophy (shrink) and gave him feelings of weakness and fatigue. Bob wasn't actually so worried about dying from his cancer but rather the remarkably high cholesterol level that had been discovered when he was diagnosed with cancer. Both Bob and Ruth were thin people with little muscle mass and lots of muscle and joint pain. When Bob was counseled about the lifestyle changes he could make to lower his cholesterol and chances of a heart attack, he was not surprised. He was well read and familiar with the elements of healthy living but just never thought that he could have high cholesterol and be at such a high risk for a heart attack. He was a thin man! Bob's misconception about his heart attack risk was shocking to him. Between the cholesterol levels and his cancer treatments he was feeling vulnerable. The idea that the cancer treatment would cause him to lose what little muscle mass he had was actually scary, which in many ways Bob found humorous, since he had never been what he describes as a "buff guy." Bob and Ruth embarked on a combined resistance and aerobic exercise program. Their goal was to exercise 3 days a week. On Monday and Friday they walked 10 to 15 minutes and did 6 resistance exercises that targeted their major muscle groups, and on Wednesday they took a longer walk around a small lake near their house. The lifestyle change took several weeks to get used to. At first, neither of them could imagine how they could fit 30 minutes of exercise into their busy schedules, but over time they found that by keeping to a regular day and time schedule they were more successful at reaching their weekly exercise goals. They were also glad that they had each other to exercise with, because when one of them didn't have the get-up-and-go to exercise, the other did. So they kept each other on target to reach their weekly exercise goal.

After 8 weeks of their exercise program, Bob's cholesterol level was lower and he began to notice that small definitions of muscle were showing in his arms that "hadn't been there before." Both Bob and his wife were surprised to find that they were experiencing fewer back and joint pains, because their muscles were getting stronger and they weren't sitting as much. They were delighted to be enjoying all of these benefits from only 30 to 45 minutes of exercise a few days a week. Now they are both regular exercisers with the goal of slowing down the aging process and doing what they can to ward off preventable conditions such as high cholesterol and high blood pressure, and of course preventing some of the muscle wasting associated with Bob's cancer treatment.

SOME BASICS OF RESISTANCE EXERCISE

A most basic and important principle of resistance exercise is to take at least 48 hours (every other day) of rest between workouts. This permits the muscles to recover and avoids the potential for injury. This rest principle is particularly important as we age and our muscles need more time to recover from the stresses imposed by resistance exercise. During your 48 hours of rest, you can safely engage in aerobic activities, such as walking or swimming, just not resistance exercises.

With any weight lifting or resistance exercises you always want to start working the largest muscles first and move to smaller and smaller muscle groups as your exercise period begins to wind down. This means starting with exercises that work the chest, such as bench press or incline dumbbell press. Leg exercises should start with lunges, squats, or leg presses. These are all exercises that work the quadriceps (front of thigh), hamstrings (back of thigh), and gluteus (buttocks). From there, start working the upper body muscles, focusing on the back, shoulders, biceps, and triceps. Lower body work should progress to focusing on specific individual muscles, such as the hamstrings, gluteus, abductors (the outside of your thigh and hip), adductors (inner muscles of your thigh), and calves.

Depending on your exercise goals and the number of days you plan on doing resistance exercises, you may want to alternate exercises between upper and lower body during your resistance exercise workout. However, some weight-training experts recommend devoting one day to focusing only on your upper body and another day on your lower body. It has always been my preference to alternate upper and lower body exercises during my resistance exercise workout. When I alternate between upper and lower body exercises, I can complete my workout in a shorter period of time because I don't need to spend a lot of time resting between sets. For example, I may do a set of chest presses and then walk over and do a set of squats or lunges, and then do another set of chest presses without stopping. By alternating between arm and leg exercises I also enjoy the benefits of a more aerobic workout; that is, my heart rate is elevated a little more because I'm not sitting around resting between each set of exercises. And lastly, by alternating between upper and lower body exercise, I don't think I get as tired. Now, if I were a body builder or power lifter, which I certainly am not, really exhausting my muscles would be optimal for faster muscle growth and strength. However, since the majority of us are not doing resistance exercises to look like Charles Atlas, following a more moderate approach of 2 days a week of resistance exercise should be sufficient not only to see strength gains but also to reap the health benefits.

DEVELOPING CORE STRENGTH

"Standing tall and strong" is a key concept of the Cancer Fitness resistance exercise program and refers to developing core strength. Core strength involves the muscles in your back, abdomen, and hips. These muscles are critical to supporting your skeleton and maintaining the proper body alignment and strength to complete everyday activities comfortably and free of pain. Weakness or muscle imbalance in your core muscles can lead to neck, back, pelvic, hip, and knee pain. Spend a few seconds before each exercise to think about "standing tall and strong" by elongating your spine, holding your shoulders back and down, contracting your abdomen and using your hips to keep you well balanced. If you make a conscious effort to stand tall and strong before you begin each exercise, it will become a habit and you will find that you are able to concentrate more on the exercise and less on your stance. Another key to healthful resistance exercise is breathing slowly, deeply, and evenly. As you perform each exercise, think about standing tall and strong and using your core muscles to provide a solid base or foundation for all of your exercises. If your core muscles are strong you will experience less pain and feel more comfortable standing and sitting for long periods of time.

FOCUS ON CORRECT FORM

Throughout this book I have emphasized the importance of doing the exercises correctly and focusing on the quality, not the quantity, of your exercise, whether the exercise is aerobic or resistance. More is not better: proper form is what's optimal. When you are doing resistance exercises, using the correct form is critical to preventing injury and benefiting from the exercise. If you are not using resistance bands, be sure you stay within your limits—don't become overly zealous or competitive and lift more weight than you are capable of. The following are some basic rules about how to learn and maintain the correct form.

1. *Do it right.* Make sure you understand the proper stance and way to hold the band or weight. Read about the proper form, or have someone show you and help you to do the exercises correctly. Have an understanding of which muscle group(s) the exercise is intended to target, and concentrate on using that muscle group when you do the exercise. Feel the muscle contract. Are you using other muscles? Performing more repetitions with incorrect or

sloppy form doesn't stimulate the muscles effectively and will not yield optimal results.

2. *Keep it light.* When you are learning a new exercise keep the resistance or weight light. Remember rule 1: Do it right. If you are struggling with a weight, you cannot concentrate on *feeling* the movement and how your muscles are working. Learn to perform the technique correctly before you increase your resistance.

3. *Look at yourself.* Yep, get in front of the mirror and check your form. Weight lifters aren't all that vain. There's a reason to watch yourself in the mirror. Look at yourself and check to see that you are beginning each exercise by standing tall and strong. Is your movement smooth? Are you moving the weight or band through the full range of motion?

4. *Ask for help.* If after practicing the exercise with a light weight and watching yourself in the mirror you still feel awkward or you just want to make sure you are doing the exercise correctly, ask your training partner to help, or if available, ask a trainer or physical therapist to check on your form. Most people in a gym setting don't want to take the risk of offending you and will not take the time to point out that your form is incorrect. If you think you aren't doing an exercise correctly, don't waste time doing the exercise or risk an injury; wait to do the exercise another time after you have gotten help to learn the correct form.

5. *Select the right resistance or weight.* To begin, realize that everything is relative to you and your strength

and that you may have some muscles that are very strong and others that are weak. What is a light weight to you may be impossibly heavy for your friend. This is a critical component of resistance exercise that is often misunderstood. Generally I see women lifting weights that are too light and men trying to move weight far too heavy for their strength. So, how do you decide what is heavy, moderate, or light? Use these general definitions:

Heavy is a weight or resistance band that you can correctly lift only 5 to 8 times.

Moderate is a weight or resistance band that you can correctly lift 8 to 10 times.

Light is a weight or resistance band that you can lift correctly 12 to 15 times.

6. *Don't be a hotshot.* Your number one goal is to exercise safely and effectively. Attempting to lift more weight than you have the strength to handle can lead to serious injury. It's okay to push yourself, but remember it takes time, persistence, and patience to develop your strength.

PRINCIPLES OF TRAINING

Just as in developing an aerobic exercise program, you need to have an understanding of how to exercise in cycles. A delightful benefit of resistance exercise is that you can see the improvements in your strength rapidly, especially when you first start. Your microcycles will show increases in strength quickly. Over time, however, what you may notice is that the gains in your strength building begin to plateau. Often this happens when you have worked hard for a series of weeks and your body needs a period of rest. As with aerobic exercise programs, rest is a critical component of a successful resistance exercise program. You need to structure your resistance exercise program to include a recovery week. Think of your resistance exercise plan as having periods of moderate or hard work and then recovery work. Does this sound like a mesocycle? It should. Weight lifters break their training up into cycles just like aerobic exercisers.

What do you do during a recovery week? Keep lifting your weights or using your bands, but use a slightly lighter weight and reduce the number of repetitions and sets. Use the recovery week to think about your form and technique. So often when we are struggling to lift a little more weight or do two more repetitions, our form begins to fall apart and we start to compensate and cheat by using other muscles so that we can move the weight those extra times. During your recovery period, move the weight slowly, think about going through the complete range of motion, and focus only on using the muscle you are working. Keep your face relaxed, avoid the animal-like grunting, and concentrate only on that one muscle or muscle group and how the muscle feels. Remember, the quality of your exercise is far more important than the quantity. Doing 4 repetitions correctly is better than 10 done incorrectly.

COMBINING AEROBIC AND RESISTANCE EXERCISE PROGRAMS

If you are interested in combining resistance exercise with your aerobic plan, there are several ways to achieve this goal successfully. One of your decisions is time related. Would you rather devote more days to exercise or more time in one day? One option is to alternate aerobic and resistance exercise days, thereby exercising more often during the week. So, your week may include aerobic exercise on Monday, Wednesday, and Friday and resistance exercise on Tuesday and Thursday. Alternatively, you could do your aerobic exercise three days a week and on two of those days, after your aerobic exercise, do your resistance exercise. A combined exercise program will give you the most all-around benefits from exercise—strength, endurance, tone, shapeliness, and improved health and wellness.

BULKING VERSUS SCULPTING

The inevitable question is, how many repetitions and sets should I do? There are a few questions you need to answer before we can come to a conclusion. Are you doing resistance exercises to regain some of the strength you lost during your illness? To improve your general health? To develop a more sculpted-looking body? To get bigger muscles? If regaining your strength is your goal, focus on completing two or three sets of 8 to 10 repetitions. The instructions in the Cancer Fitness resistance exercise program (Chapter 9) can help you make decisions about when to increase your resistance or weight. For general health purposes, the American College of Sports Medicine (ACSM) recommends performing one set of 8 to 10 repetitions using moderate to heavy weight at least two times a week to maintain strength and improve your health. The ACSM suggests doing resistance exercises that focus on the major muscle groups.

For a more sculpted body with longer-looking muscles, you will need to take a more endurance type of approach and focus on increasing the number of repetitions. Of course, to increase your repetitions you will have to reduce the amount of weight you are lifting or the resistance on the bands. When I first started doing this type of exercise, I was shocked by how little weight I could lift and still complete the exercises. If you decide to select this approach to resistance exercise, try to do two or three sets of 18 to 22 repetitions. Beware, however: your muscles will scream when you first start this type of resistance exercise. Realize that by working toward a more sculpted body you will not develop the power of someone lifting more weights and doing fewer repetitions, but your muscles will become well defined and have good endurance.

If bigger muscles are your goal, then you should focus on doing fewer repetitions and lifting heavier weights. A popular approach to developing strength and muscle mass is to use a pyramid approach. This means doing perhaps 10 repetitions using a light weight, then increasing the weight and decreasing the number of repetitions with each subsequent set of lifts. The last set of lifts you may be moving a weight that you can only lift one or two times. You may need a friend to spot you so you don't get hurt. I don't recommend this approach to weight lifting for most people unless you are aiming to get strong again and return to competitive sport or rebuild a muscular physique.

If you are simply looking at resistance exercise as a way to improve your health during and following treatment, I recommend following an integrated resistance and aerobic exercise program. To start, try the Cancer Fitness programs. If you want to do more or different exercises, then follow the guidelines in this chapter and the previous one to develop an efficient and effective exercise program to suite your individual needs and goals.

DON'T GET STUCK IN A RUT

Do different exercises. Often we start doing 6 or 8 exercises and keep doing the same thing every time we work out. What happens when you do this is that your muscles become very strong for that particular movement, but what you want is muscles that are useful in a variety of different positions. After all, our everyday life is fluid and isn't limited to one motion. To build functional and useful muscle strength you need to vary your workout. Do lunges and walking lunges, biceps curls standing up and sitting down. Both these exercises are basically the same, but the change in position helps us to strengthen our muscles in slightly different angles, thereby giving us more functional strength.

It's easy to get stuck in the same exercise pattern. You get used to doing "your" exercises, and you know how to do them and how to set up the equipment correctly. Often we get stuck in a rut because we don't know other exercises that will effectively target the same muscle group but through a different movement. This book shows you some exercises, but there are many more that you can do to strengthen your body in functional, fun, and creative ways. It may be helpful for you to work with a trainer in your area or to read a few books on weight-training exercises.

SICK DAYS AND OVERTRAINING

Resistance exercise is no different from aerobic exercise. If you are sick, take time off to let your body heal and rejuvenate. If you work yourself so hard that you become overtrained, take a few days off, or if you are so committed to your exercise program that taking a day off scares you, then cut the amount of weight you lift by at least 30 percent and also reduce the number of repetitions and sets. Spend this recovery time focusing on your form. It is more difficult to become overtrained simply through resistance exercise than aerobic exercise, assuming that you build in periods of recovery. The sensations of overtraining you are most likely to encounter from resistance training include increasing muscle soreness and fatigue. A feeling that I often associate with being overtrained is emptiness in my muscles. My muscles feel drained of their energy and as if the exercise takes far more oomph to do than it usually does. Taking a few days off and concentrating on eating a diet high in carbohydrates tends to get me right back on track. Again, rest is the best way to recover from illness and overtraining. Take a few days off to let your muscles recover. If you really feel compelled to exercise, then go for an easy walk.

SUMMARY

Developing and maintaining a strong, active, stable, and resilient body can only enhance the quality of your life as you age. Clearly, we can't stop the clock, but we certainly can delay some of the effects of the aging process on our bodies. If you are going to develop your own progressive resistance exercise program, be sure the plan includes periods of rest and recovery, and give yourself the time to progress slowly at your own pace. Your plan should include different exercises to work your muscles in a variety of ways that target all the major muscles of the body. Developing and maintaining both strong core musculature (in order to stand tall and strong) and well balanced muscle strength in your major muscle groups are important for maintaining functional ability and independence, and for ensuring your ability to participate actively with family and friends as you go through different phases of your cancer treatment—to say nothing of the eternal quest for the fountain of youth.

REVIEW POINTS

- Don't start resistance exercises until you are at least 4 weeks past surgery, unless your doctor gives you permission sooner.
- Start slowly and expect to progress slowly.
- Notice any unusual changes in your body. If you are at risk for or have lymphedema, measure the girth of your arm or leg every morning. If you notice swelling, contact your health care team or your physical therapist. It is important to intervene early.
- Before beginning an exercise, think about standing tall and strong, relaxing your face, and breathing deeply.
- Do each exercise slowly, and work your muscles through the full range of motion. If you find your-

self leaning, compensate by using other muscles, or find other ways to cheat to lift more weight, then stop the exercise and reduce the weight or resistance. Correct form is your number one priority.

CHAPTER 9

CANCER FITNESS

RESISTANCE EXERCISE PROGRAM

The resistance exercise program in this chapter can be performed alone or in combination with an aerobics exercise program. I have used it both ways in my exercise studies. It is straightforward and should be completed in 30 minutes or less. If you were to select only one exercise program to follow, I would recommend starting the aerobic exercise program (Chapter 6), because aerobic exercise confers the greatest health benefits in the long term and will keep you functionally able during and following treatment. However, the Cancer Fitness resistance exercise program (Table 6) is ideal if you are confined to bed, have muscle weakness that needs to be remedied, or simply want to get stronger.

Table 6. Cancer Fitness Resistance Exercise Program

How often do I need to do the resistance exercise?
Two or 3 days a week, alternating between exercise program A and B. Don't do the exercises 2 days in a row.

Does it matter if I do all the arm or leg exercises at once? Yes! Alternate between lower and upper body exercise to give each muscle group a rest between exercises. This will help you to gain benefits from the exercises. Start working your large muscle groups (thighs, back, and chest) and then move to smaller ones (e.g., calves, biceps, and triceps).

How hard do I have to do the resistance exercise? Exercise within your ability and comfort. Move the elastic band or weight to a count of 3, and release the band to a count of 3. There should be even tension on the band throughout the movement. Be sure you control the band back to the resting position. Don't let the band snap back. Remember to concentrate on your form and posture. Hold your core muscles (abdomen, back, and hips) tight, and breathe with each exercise.

What are repetitions and sets? This is strength-training lingo. A complete movement (lifting the weight or band up and returning to your starting position) is called one repetition. So, if you are doing 8 repetitions, you would do the complete exercise movement 8 times. If you did 8 repetitions, rested for a few minutes, and did another 8 repetitions, you would have completed 2 sets. In this program a set is 8 to 12 repetitions.

How many repetitions and sets of each exercise should I do? To maintain and build your strength, do 2 or 3 sets of 8 to 12 repetitions of each exercise. If after doing this for four months you want to increase your muscular endurance, increase the repetitions to 15 to 20 and lower your resistance or weight by about 25 percent. If you are using a band to do the exercise, you may want to go down to the next band, one with less resistance. However, if you want to increase your strength progressively, you will need to continue to increase the amount of resistance or weight you are moving: continue doing 2 to 3 sets of 8 repetitions.

Can I do the resistance exercises two days in a row? No, this isn't a good idea. Your muscles need time to recover. If you do resistance exercises two days in a row and work the same muscle groups, you will get very sore and achy and limit the progress you can make.

Remember and write down: In your exercise log (see Chapter 4), keep track of how long you exercised (number of minutes), the exercise you did (A or B), the color of the elastic band or the amount of weight you used, and the number of repetitions and sets you completed.

How do I know when to change to a different resistance band or weight? When you can complete, using good form, 3 sets of 12 repetitions, you are ready to increase to the next color resistance band or increase your weight by 2 to 5 pounds. If you only have weights that increase in 5-pound increments and that is too large an increase, then maintain the same weight but increase the number of repetitions you do to 15. When you can complete 3 sets or 15 repetitions, then you will have the strength to increase the weight. If you can only complete one or two sets of 8 repetitions at the new weight, then complete the final sets at the old weight.

Resistance exercise can be done with stretchy tubing like Thera-Bands or with weights either by using machines in a gym or free weights (e.g., dumbbells or hand weights). Elastic exercise bands are inexpensive, easy to use at home, compact, and lightweight. They come in different colors, which represent different thicknesses or degrees of resistance. The only challenge with the elastic bands is that initially you will need to spend some time determining where and how best to secure them for each exercise, which can be different depending on your house and furniture. The directions for the different exercises should give you some idea of how best to use the bands in your situation.

If you use weights it doesn't matter whether you use machines or free weights. Exercise machines tend to help you maintain proper form, reduce the risk from injury, and allow you to lift greater weight. However, free weights help you improve your balance, coordination, and muscle balance. Free weights are fairly inexpensive and are practical to use at home. I prefer to use a combination of free weights and bands when I work out because they help to keep my muscles equally strong on both sides of my body, and I can do my workouts at home.

For safety reasons, I urge you to avoid using homemade weights devised out of milk jugs, empty detergent containers, or cans of food loaded into bags. These items are not designed for weight training and could be unsafe by altering your balance or gait. If you are looking for a way to economize, buy a set of exercise elastic bands (e.g., Thera-Bands) or just a few weights that you are most likely to use, or share weights with a friend. Your safety is what's most important.

When you start resistance exercises begin with light weights. I mean embarrassingly light weight. You should be able to complete easily, using good form, 12 repetitions without straining. If you start off lifting weight that is too heavy, you may not be able to complete the workout, or worse, your muscles may become incredibly sore in the day or two following the workout, which may make you feel discouraged. Take your time. Your body is responsive and will adapt to lifting the weights. Don't push it. If the exercise is too hard, back the weight or resistance down to a degree at which you can complete the exercise using good form and without hurting yourself. When you first begin exercising you may feel some muscle soreness, but this is normal. You are making your muscles work more than they are accustomed to, but as you become stronger you can push yourself harder.

Breathing is the most natural thing, but sometimes when we lift weights or pull on elastic bands we concentrate so much on good form or completing the exercise that we forget to breathe. Remember, breathe in through your nose and out through your mouth. Scan your body for tension: relax your face muscles, keep your jaw relaxed so you won't clench your teeth, and think about good posture with relaxed shoulders. Concentrate on using only the muscle group you are strengthening.

After slowly starting a resistance exercise program and doing so for the past 3 weeks, I'm at the point where if I don't get my regular exercise I get grumpy. It's like a drug—it makes me feel so much better about everything.

—Ivan, 49 years old, a bladder cancer patient

ADDITIONAL NOTES BEFORE YOU START THE RESISTANCE EXERCISES

Before you begin any of these exercises, take a moment to think about standing tall and strong. What exactly does this mean? Stand up straight with your stomach and center area pulled in, relax your shoulders, and think about using the muscles in the core of your body (trunk and buttocks) to stabilize you and help you to maintain good form. By being mindful of standing tall and strong you will not only benefit more from each individual exercise but also build your core strength, which will help with your balance and physical endurance.

When you first begin exercising with Thera-bands or an equivalent band, be patient. It takes some time to learn the optimal way or place to secure them for each exercise. The bands are easiest to use if you have the ankle assist, handle, and door anchor accessories. However, if you do not purchase these you can still do the exercises by making a knot at the end of each band to use for the arm exercises, tying the ends of the band together for the ankle and leg exercises and tying a knot in the center of the band to put over the door for those exercise. You will undoubtedly need different band tensions for your arm and leg exercises, which will make all this tying and positioning easier.

For the exercises that can be done easily with free weights, I've explained how to do the exercise below the band instructions.

RESISTANCE EXERCISE PROGRAM A

Squats

Stand on the center of the band. Place your feet hip width apart and bring the band up to shoulder level. Slowly bend your knees until they are at a 45 degree angle. Keep your knees behind your toes. Slowly push yourself back up to the starting position. Repeat.

Free weights: These can be done with either dumbbell or bands. If you use dumbbells, hold one in each hand at your sides and keep the weight there throughout the exercise. Bend your knees 45 degrees, keeping your knees behind your toes, and slowly return to the start position.

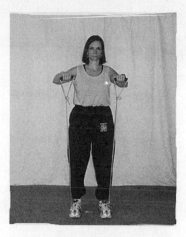

FIGURE 11
Starting position for squat.

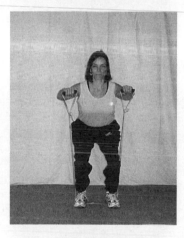

FIGURE 12
Keep knees behind toes.

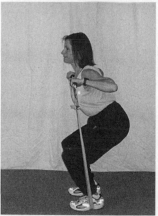

FIGURE 13
Side view of squat.

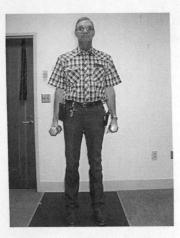

FIGURE 14
Starting position for dumbbell squats.

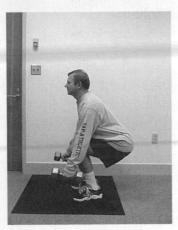

FIGURE 15
Ending position for dumbbell squats. Keep knees behind toes, and work to get thigh parallel to the floor.

Lat Pull-Downs

Secure the middle of the band to the top of the door. As you face the door, grasp the ends of the tubing with your palms facing down. Stand about 2 feet from the door. Pull the bands toward your shoulders. Slowly control the band back to your starting position. Repeat.

Lat pull–downs can be done on a machine if you exercise in a gym.

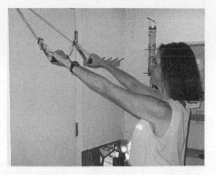

FIGURE 16
Starting position.

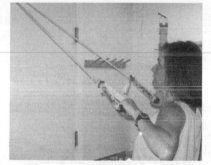

FIGURE 17
Final position.

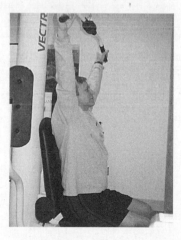

FIGURE 18
Starting position for lat pull-downs on a machine.

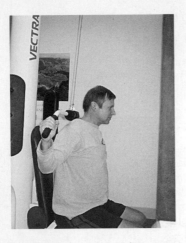

FIGURE 19
Ending position for lat pull-downs.

Leg Extensions

Loop the band around a sturdy object, like a leg of a couch, heavy chair, or table leg, or wedge it in the bottom of the door. Place the band around your leg, and step out forward so that the band is slightly taut against your leg. With your back to the table or door, slowly extend your leg straight out in front of you and slowly return to your original standing position. Use your core muscles to maintain an upright position. If you find yourself leaning in the opposite direction, hold on to something to help you balance and lighten up the tension on the band. Repeat on the starting leg and then continue exercises on the opposite leg.

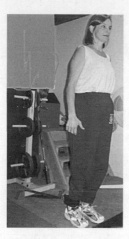

FIGURE 20
Starting position.

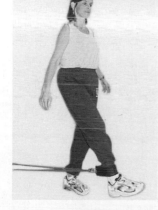

FIGURE 21
Final position of leg extension.

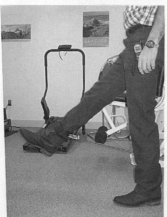

FIGURE 22
Final position of leg extension.

Flies

Use the same setup as for the lat pull-downs. For this exercise, stand with your back to the door. Grasp the bands with your arms outstretched and parallel to the floor and your palms facing forward. Slowly pull the band to bring your hands in front of you. Keep your arms straight. Slowly control the band back to your starting position and repeat.

Free weights: Lie on your back on a weight bench. Holding the weight in either hand, extend your arms out to the side. Your palms should be facing the ceiling. Keeping your arms straight, bring the weight directly over your body. Control your arms back to the starting position. Repeat.

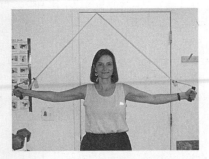

FIGURE 23
Starting position.

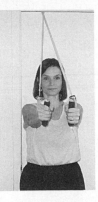

FIGURE 24
Ending position.

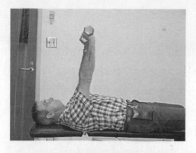

FIGURE 25
Dumbbell starting position with weight held directly above you.

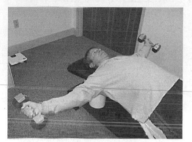

FIGURE 26
Ending position.

Adduction Side Kicks

Use the setup for the leg extensions. Stand with the door or table at your side and the ankle of your inside leg in the loop. Stand on the outside leg, hold yourself tall and strong, and pull the band across your other leg. Slowly let the band back to your starting position. Repeat. Turn around and repeat the exercise on the other leg.

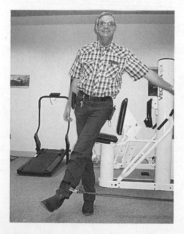

FIGURE 27
Adduction: pull the band across your body.

Bicep Curl

Stand on one end of the band, and hold the other end in your hand. Your palm should be facing up. Keep your wrist straight as you curl your arm up to your shoulder. Control the band back to the starting position, and repeat the exercise. Remember to do the exercise with your other arm, too.

Free weights: Hold a weight in each hand and follow the directions above.

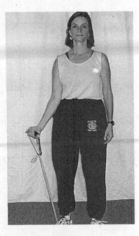

FIGURE 28
Starting position for biceps curl.

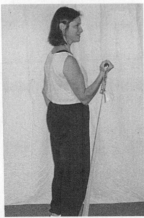

FIGURE 29
Ending position for biceps curl.

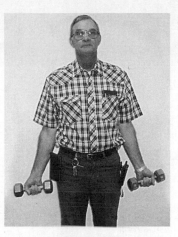

FIGURE 30
Starting position for dumbbell bicep curls.

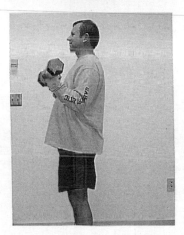

FIGURE 31
Ending position for biceps curls.

Abduction Side Kicks

Use the setup for the leg extensions. Stand with the door or table at your side and the ankle of your inside leg in the loop. Stand on the inside leg, hold yourself tall and strong, and pull the band out to the side, lifting your leg about 3 inches off the floor. Keep your leg straight. Slowly let the band back to your starting position. Repeat. Turn around and repeat the exercise working the other leg.

Hold on to a chair, couch, or table to stabilize yourself so that you can concentrate on doing the motion correctly.

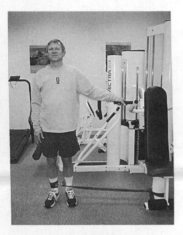

FIGURE 32
Starting position for abduction.

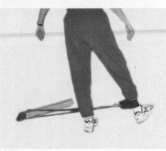

FIGURE 33
Abduction: pull the band away from your body.

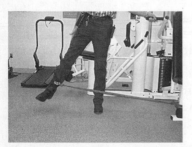

FIGURE 34
Front view of abduction.

RESISTANCE EXERCISE PROGRAM B

Lunges

Secure the band in the door slightly above your head. Face away from the door, and grasp the band on either end. Hold the ends at chest level with your palms facing forward. Step forward on one leg, and bend that knee until your thigh is parallel to the floor. Keep your knees behind your toes. Push yourself back to your starting position and step forward with the other leg to begin the exercise again.

Free weights: Hold a weight in either hand at your side. Relax your shoulders, and step forward with one leg and follow the directions above.

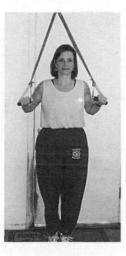

FIGURE 35
Starting position for lunges.

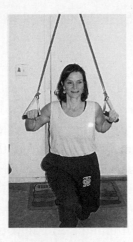

FIGURE 36
Front view of lunge.

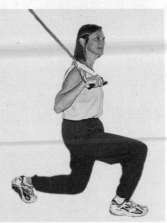

FIGURE 37
Side view of lunge. Notice how her thigh is parallel to the floor.

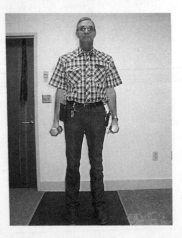

FIGURE 38
Starting position for lunge. Step straight forward.

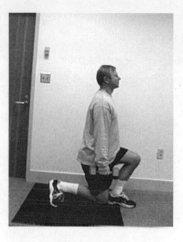

FIGURE 39
Ending lunge position, keeping knee behind toes.

Chest Press

Use the band setup for the lunges. Stand facing away from the door. Hold the band at your armpit level with your palms toward the floor. Push the band straight out in front of you. Extend your arms all the way out. Slowly control the band back to your starting position. Repeat.

Free weights: Lie on your back on a bench. Start with a weight in each hand and your hands at armpit level with your palms facing the ceiling. Push the weight straight up over your body until your arms are straight. Slowly lower the weight back to the starting position and repeat.

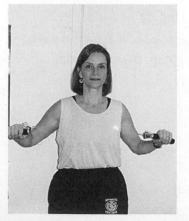

FIGURE 40
Starting position.

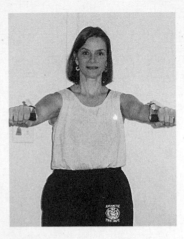

FIGURE 41

Arms extended straight out in front of body.

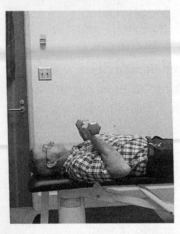

FIGURE 42

Hold your arms shoulder width apart, and start the exercise with the dumbbells just above your shoulders.

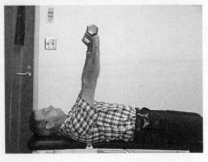

FIGURE 43

Ending position. Push the weight straight up over your body.

Hamstring Curls

Use the setup for the leg extensions. Stand facing the door or table. With the band around your ankle, pull the heel of your foot up toward your buttock. Remember to stand tall and strong. Hold on to something if you find yourself leaning forward. Control the bend back to your starting position. Repeat. Then continue the exercise on the opposite leg.

Hamstring curls can be done on a machine if you exercise in a gym.

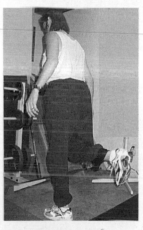

FIGURE 44
Hamstring curl. Curl leg up to at least 45 degrees.

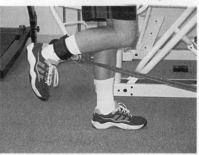

FIGURE 45
Curl leg up to at least 45 degrees.

Bent Rowing

Stand on the band and bend forward about 45 degrees. Hold the band in one hand with your palm facing your body. Slowly pull the band up to your armpit, and return to your starting position. Lean on a chair or other object to keep your balance. Think about holding your core muscles strong and keeping your back long and straight. Remember to do this exercise with your other arm.

Free weights: Hold a weight in one hand and follow the directions above.

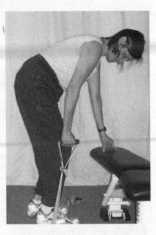

FIGURE 46
Starting position. Keep back flat.

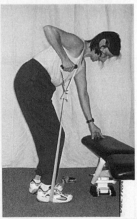

FIGURE 47
Ending bent rowing position.

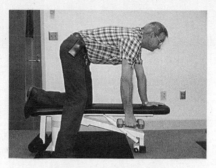

FIGURE 48
Starting position for dumbbell bent rowing. Nice flat back to start.

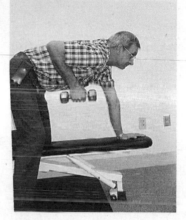

FIGURE 49
Ending position of dumbbell bent rowing.

Hip Extension

Use the setup for the leg extensions. Stand facing the door or other object that is securing the band. Place your ankle inside the loop. Stand on the opposite leg, hold yourself tall and strong, and pull the band straight back, lifting your leg about 3 inches off the floor. Keep your leg straight. Slowly let the band back to your starting position. Repeat. Do the exercise working the other leg, too.

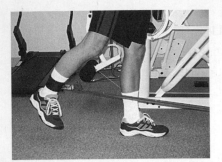

FIGURE 50

Pull the band straight back. Concentrate on keeping your hips square: that is, don't let them roll back to help you move the band back.

Tricep Press

Stand on one end of the band, and hold the other end in your hand. Bend your arm back over your shoulder as though you were trying to scratch your head. Your palm should be facing just behind your ear. Keep your wrist straight as you extend your arm straight. Control the band back to the starting position, and repeat the exercise. Remember to do the exercise with your other arm, too.

Free weights: Hold a weight in one hand and follow the directions above.

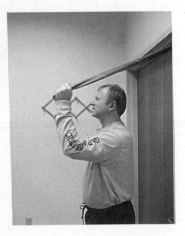

FIGURE 51

Starting position for tricep press.

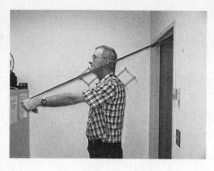

FIGURE 52

Ending position with arm fully extended.

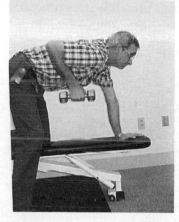

FIGURE 53

Start with the weight curled all the way up to your shoulder.

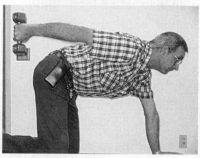

FIGURE 54

Extend the weight straight back.

COMBINING THE AEROBIC AND RESISTANCE EXERCISE PROGRAMS

There are several ways to combine aerobic and resistance exercise programs. You could exercise 3 days a week by combining aerobic and resistance workouts or as many as 5 or 6 days a week by doing aerobic exercise one day and resistance exercise the next. If you choose to exercise 3 days a week, do your aerobic exercise first so that you can get a good warmup before the resistance exercise. A benefit of doing the aerobic exercise first is that your muscles aren't tired from the resistance exercises. If you prefer to alternate aerobic and resistance exercise over 5 or 6 days, that's fine, but remember, do not do resistance exercises 2 days in row. Let your muscles recover by doing an aerobic exercise or taking the day off.

KEEPING AN EXERCISE LOG

You don't have to keep a log, but it sure helps. An exercise log helps you to see your improvements over time, determine when to start increasing your exercise program, and even see patterns that have successfully helped you to build your body up for a hike or other event. A log doesn't take a lot of time to complete. It will help you to analyze your past mistakes, when you may have increased your exercise intensity too much, as well as your successes.

After I set my first 24-hour bicycling distance record, I looked back in my logs to see how I did it. The information in my log was the "recipe" for my success, and before future 24-hour records I would follow the same basic recipe but would increase the intensity of my training, because I was another year stronger and smarter. That is, I knew how to recognize when I was getting overtrained and would generally back off and rest before I fell into the overtraining abyss. Review the exercise logs in Chapter 4. You may want to use one of these forms, create your own, or use a wall calendar.

SUMMARY

Following one of the Cancer Fitness exercise programs will help you to see steady physical and emotional improvements and long-term health benefits. The exercise plans have been tested on hundreds of patients with positive outcomes. For you to see steady improvement it will be necessary to find a balance between exercising at different intensities and resting. When you keep a log of the exercise you do, it is easy to see the rapid progress you are making that builds on your previous activities. A keen awareness of your body's need for rest, a healthy low-fat diet, and the motivating techniques presented in previous and future chapters are vital to integrating exercise into your daily life. Combined with the suggestions in this book, realistic goal setting, personal commitment, and hard work, not only can you achieve your goals, but you can also exceed your personal preconceived limits.

CHAPTER 10

THE UNTHINKABLE:
RECURRENT CANCER AND EXERCISE

In all my years of work in oncology, I've never met a patient
or a long-term survivor who has not experienced emotional pain and fear of recurrence for months and even years
after the completion of treatment. Every ache and pain is
translated into worry about recurrence of cancer. The most
common, dreaded, and overwhelming fear, recurrence of
cancer and metastatic disease, is one that we have the strength
to work through and live with or beyond. For many patients,
recurrence is not only a shock but is far more frightening
than the original diagnosis. Gathering the emotional and
spiritual strength to cope with recurrence and uncertainty is
enormous.

The common course of advanced cancers varies widely
by type of disease and an individual's response to treatment,
which can be unpredictable. The good news is that many
cancer survivors have experienced multiple recurrences and
still achieved complete remission, and others with metastatic

disease go on to enjoy many productive years with their disease in control. Although cancer may leave our bodies with scars and deformities, exercise can help prevent the physical declines that sap the vitality from many survivors who have meaningful, dynamic lives to live. Exercise can help rebuild self-confidence, a level of trust in one's body, and an awareness of the powerful role that we play in our own physical and emotional healing. While exercise will not erase all the fears of recurrence and unpleasant memories, it does help to reduce some of the anxiety, to restore faith in your body's ability to perform "normally," and to give you a feeling of control. Exercise has a vital place in healing the soul and strengthening the body during this fragile time.

A RESEARCH AND CLINICAL PERSPECTIVE

I began this research and lifework because of my observations and experiences working with bone marrow transplant patients in the mid-1980s. Most of these patients had recurrent or metastatic disease, and over time I observed that some patients didn't seem to suffer to the same degree as the others. What was different about these patients? They were more physically active. The increased activity seemed to put them in a better mood, and they seemed more engaged with their surroundings. Some patients even insisted on making their own beds in the morning. Exercise in very small doses, even for these patients who were receiving the toughest of treatments, seemed to reduce the level of fatigue, weight change, depression, anxiety, and suffering.

There is a growing body of research on the effects of exercise during and following cancer treatment, but there is little reported about the effects of exercise in patients with recurrent or metastatic disease. Although hundreds of people with advanced cancer have participated in community exercise programs or developed their own programs, only one research study has examined the effects of exercise on patients with metastatic cancer. This study reinforced the findings from studies with patients who have earlier stages of disease—the patients got stronger, fitter, and faster while enjoying less anxiety and better emotional health. My research has primarily studied patients with earlier stages of cancer, but I follow my patients for a long period of time, and unfortunately some patients have developed recurrent or more advanced disease. What I have observed in my research and in my clinical practice is that exercise is beneficial and safe for patients with advanced disease. Exercise not only helps reduce anxiety and depression, but also maintains muscle strength so that you don't become too debilitated to participate in those important activities you really want to live for. Sustaining your physical strength may be the most important aspect of exercise for people with advanced cancer who want to continue being involved in their life pursuits.

GOALS

Now is the time to reevaluate your life and make those honest decisions about how you want to spend your time and live. Some people want to take a big trip and see the world, others seek to conquer a physical challenge like climbing a mountain peak, and still others want to stick close to home and be with family or immerse themselves in their work.

There is no right or wrong choice; the correct choice is deciding what is important to you in living life fully.

Although there are some special precautions you should be aware of when you exercise, the basic prescription and methods for getting or staying strong are the same as those discussed in previous chapters. You will want to build slowly and steadily. If you have been exercising and are now confronted with this new life challenge, cut the intensity and duration of your workout in half and see how you do. Because of the recurrence, you will probably receive a different treatment regimen than you did originally. Even though you are familiar with the basic routine, you will need to see how you tolerate the first cycle of chemotherapy. You may need to learn how to manage new side effects, which may be specific to the type of chemotherapy you are receiving. Once you see how your body responds to the treatment, then you can gradually start to increase your exercise duration and intensity. Many people find that with each recurrence they become more adept at managing their side effects and anticipating what to expect, but your body can react in unexpected ways to each type of treatment you receive, which is why I urge you to proceed slowly with your exercise program.

THE STRENGTH TO KEEP GOING

Martha was a 40-ish woman with breast cancer with whom I became good friends. Over the course of many years, she endured multiple recurrences and eventually developed lung, liver, and brain metastasis. She had many life dreams and goals of travels as well as activities she wanted to continue to pursue. One of her favorite activities was taking the dogs to the park. For many months we would take long walks with our dogs. As Martha's disease progressed or on days when she felt particularly tired, she would push a walker with a seat attachment so she could rest. We continued to take long walks and Martha maintained her strength, but when she began to have problems with balance and heat intolerance, she decided that a wheelchair would give her more freedom. Much to her surprise, the wheelchair permitted us to go on longer excursions and gave us more freedom because Martha knew I could always push her home. Martha's strength and independence allowed her to live independently and continue doing the activities she loved much longer than if she had gone home and curled up on the couch. Martha told me, "exercise helps me to keep a strong hold on life, and keep going. I can't stop. I wish exercise was just part of everyone's treatment plan, it's the best medicine there is."

SPECIAL EXERCISE CONSIDERATIONS

There are a few precautions one should take before beginning or resuming exercise with a new recurrence or metastatic disease, and they focus on whether you have metastasis to your bones, lungs, central nervous system, or brain. If you have bony lesions from a cancer that has metastasized to the bone, you need to consult with your physician about activities that are safe to participate in. If there is a risk that you could fracture a bone from jumping or running, it would be better to know this in advance and focus your activities on non–weight-bearing sports, such as swimming, using a stationary bicycle, or rowing.

Lung involvement, whether it is from lung cancer or metastasis of the cancer to your lung, can cause problems with breathing, which may make exercise much more challenging. Plan your exercise so that you have time to rest and catch your breath and ideally a place to sit down if you need to. With lung metastasis, it is important to start your exercise program very slowly and gradually progress. If you start off doing too much too soon and advance too quickly, you may soon become very frustrated, tired, and disgusted. Go slowly, pace yourself so you don't become too breathless, and be patient with your progress.

If you have central nervous system metastasis or lesions in the brain, you may have problems with dizziness, vision changes, and problems with heat intolerance. Dizziness or vision changes may have been the symptom that prompted the discovery of your cancer or recurrence. Fear not, there is no reason to stop being physically active. You just need some guidance to know what is safe to do before you exercise.

Nothing could be worse than having a serious injury from working hard to keep yourself healthy and strong. If your physician does not know what type of exercise to recommend, advocate for yourself and ask for a referral to see someone in physical therapy or in rehabilitation medicine. The last thing you want to do is to go home, become a couch potato, and let the whole situation overwhelm you simply because you don't know how to exercise safely. There are plenty of creative ways to keep yourself strong and active and living fully in the face of uncertainty.

This is a good time to review the symptom management suggestions in Chapter 3. To live the fullest life possible, you need to keep your side effects to a minimum, which means learning to interpret your symptoms, how best to manage them before they become too unbearable, and maintaining an open dialogue with your health care team to coordinate early intervention if your current side effects management plan is not working adequately.

Daniel Shapiro is a friend and was a patient who was diagnosed as an adolescent with non-Hodgkin's lymphoma. He experienced multiple relapses and underwent many courses of chemotherapy, radiotherapy, bone marrow transplant, and then more rigorous chemotherapy. His description of exercise helps us to understand how important our role is in healing our body and soul.

Exercise was the first thing I could do for myself after my bone marrow transplant. Through daily puttering in the water, and then swimming, I could experience objective improvements in my body's functioning. I could feel myself getting stronger and returning to normal. I think it also improved my mood through direct physical channels—I was a nicer person to be around after I exercised. Those habits stayed with me, I play ultimate Frisbee three times a week now and it's been ten years since I was last treated.

CHAPTER 11

REALIZING YOUR POTENTIAL

I don't think it is possible to go through cancer treatment and not be changed by it. Oddly enough, cancer is often the significant life event that one needs to commit to making important healthy lifestyle changes. If you are a patient or a survivor, exercise provides a medium to develop self-confidence, a positive self-image, and a sense of well-being to reclaim your body and your life. The inner strength that is so often learned through cancer and exercise can be a means to push beyond one's personal, self-imposed limitations, and I have seen many patients use this learning to excel in other areas of their lives that they did not think imaginable.

The tools for successful fitness and making exercise an integral part of your life can be used to accomplish other goals in your life. In my studies, I've seen patients develop a belief in themselves and their ability to overcome their treatment as they start to exercise, often exercising for the first time in their lives. These patients develop a strong sense of purpose that benefits them not only physically but also emotionally. Through goal setting, persistence, determination, and visualization, exercise may help us succeed in our personal lives in ways we did not imagine or anticipate. Achieving your best, exceeding your expectations, and reaching for the highest standards is up to you; we all have the power to choose what is important and meaningful in our lives.

Be honest with yourself as you evaluate what it is you want to do that has meaning and importance to you. Formulate a plan and the steps that you think will be necessary to reach your life goal(s), which may or may not be exercise related. However, you may find that exercise may be the path that helps you to figure out what it is that you really want to do. Often exercise gets you away from the overwhelming number of life distractions and gives you valuable contemplative time to consider life issues in a different light, and develop the self-confidence to meet those goals. Exercise may actually be a passageway for you to discover new aspects about yourself and your life, not only from a physical perspective, but also an emotional and spiritual perspective.

Often when I'm out riding my bicycle, running in the woods, or walking through a fresh snowfall with my dogs, I find myself in a lively dialogue with myself. My mind talks loudly, sometimes so loudly that I wonder if other people can hear my thoughts, sorting out problems at work, considering a new, more creative approach to working with a challenging issue, or simply daydreaming.

Dreams can become realities. As you dream and make that dream more concrete by visualizing yourself doing the activity, imagining what the scene smells like, how it feels, how you look, and all the steps that it takes to get there, soon you can begin to really see yourself achieving your dream.

Once you believe, you can achieve your dream, but with a lot of hard work.

As a child I used to dream about going on adventures, being an athlete, and riding my bicycle across the United States. It was 1976, the year of the bicentennial celebration, and my family was driving across the country following much of the bicentennial route. We spent a wonderful time exploring the Rocky Mountains, and we kept passing two young men who were riding fully loaded touring bicycles across the United States. They were not only handsome, but they appeared to be having a fantastic and unforgettable time riding through the breathtaking mountains and wide-open plains and smelling the pine trees and sweet sage and creosote of the desert. Their travels captured my imagination, and I dreamed about embarking on such an adventure. Little did I know that over 20 years later, my childhood dream would come true and I would be able to ride in 17 days from San Diego to Jacksonville Beach, Florida. It was a life challenge and a fantastic journey. My childhood daydreaming was a form of visualization. The time I spent visualizing myself getting strong and fit, and cycling over mountains, influenced me in such a way that when the time was right in my life, I was able to make the trip more than a childhood dream.

What I have learned personally and seen many of my patients learn is that exercise can positively affect all aspects or our lives. Through exercise we can learn *intensity, concentration,* and *enthusiasm,* three powerful words that are key in the pursuit of excellence, regardless of whether your life passion is overcoming cancer, succeeding in business, sports, or raising a family. Realizing your potential takes commitment, self-discipline, concentration, and inner strength. If you do not enjoy what you are doing, life becomes drudgery, and then you must stop and ask yourself why you are doing what you are doing. What is your motivation? What is the reward? Realizing your potential depends to a great extent on three things:

Intensity. Give 100 percent of yourself to your pursuit of excellence. Keep yourself fully present and focused on your passion, which will help you to stay mindful and attentive. Without this 100 percent commitment and discipline you cannot overcome the hurdles and barriers we all encounter, whether they are in sport, business, or family.

Concentration. Come to your activity, work, and life passion fully prepared to focus only on what you are doing and ready to be completely absorbed in it. When you become so absorbed in your work, or exercise, or whatever it is you are doing that the distractions and of hassles of daily life fall to the side, then you are completely present and aware in the moment—fully concentrating. Learn to leave the daily hassles and frustrations out of the way and to tune out your distractions. We all know that distractions will always be there; this is a given in life. By having a clearly formulated plan and goal, you will stay focused and motivated.

Enthusiasm. Pursue your passion with a positive attitude and outlook. Be positive and optimistic about what you are doing and supportive of others in their pursuits. Work to surround yourself with positive, affirming, and encouraging people who believe in you, your ability, and your pursuit of excellence. As you being to think and see life more positively, unexpected rewards will often begin to unfold. If you feel you are losing your laughter, spontaneity, and life passion, ask yourself what has changed. Where did the fun go? Am I doing what is really important to me? Am I doing what I think is valuable to my family and society? It's never too late to change tacts. Just open your heart and listen to what it is telling you—follow your deeper instincts, not what you think "they" want you to do.

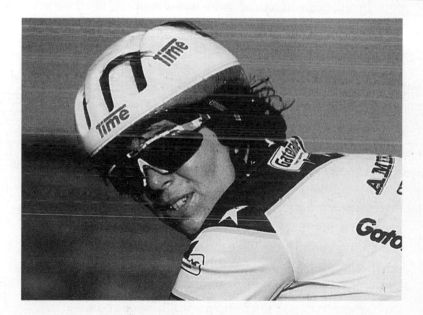

The author on the road to a world record, Homestead, Florida, May 1992.

RELAXATION

Relaxation can bring the centered calmness that is key to developing the intensity, concentration, and enthusiasm to meet your goals. Fortunately, we are not all alike and are attracted to different activities, hobbies, and vocations. We gravitate to the things that suit our nature, ability, and temperament. However, we all share the unpleasant sensations of anxiety, worry, and tension. Techniques to manage these stressful feelings can help us through difficult medical procedures, an interview for a job, or a first date. Relaxation means letting go completely of your muscle tension, focusing on your breathing, and letting your mind drift.

Relaxation is a skill that requires learning and practice but can give you a greater sensitivity and awareness of your body. An easy form of relaxation that can help you in any situation is to become aware of your breathing and focus on taking slow, deep full breaths in through your nose and out through your mouth. Feel your tension release itself with each breath. This is a technique you can use anywhere and one that can help you feel more centered at stressful times. There are many excellent books on relaxation techniques that range from progressive relaxation to meditation to autogenic training. I will not elaborate on the techniques here, but taking the time to incorporate relaxation into your life can help you to feel and become more centered and calm, which can facilitate and foster your ability to have the intensity, concentration, and energy to reach your goals.

VISUALIZATION

Much of success rests on our imagination and belief in our ability to achieve a goal. When I set out to achieve my first 24-hour cycling record, I was apprehensive, but my friend and coach Betsy King made me believe in myself. She convinced me that I could reach my goal, and she was right. Entering my doctoral program I had many uncertainties about my abilities, but my mentor supported me and repeatedly told me I could succeed. She was right, too. Even if we don't have 100 percent confidence in our ability to reach our goals, aligning ourselves with people who are successful, supportive, and reliable cheerleaders makes reaching our peak possible. These positive people in our lives help us to take the small steps that are essential for reaching out goals.

Seeing yourself reaching your goal is critical, whether it is walking to the end of the block, running a mile, or making a big presentation. Athletes, actors, and many other people use visual imagery to improve their performance. When I coach bicyclists I tell my students to visualize themselves sprinting or climbing a hill using the correct form, controlling their breathing, and feeling relaxed. I have used visualization to win races, prepare before a big presentation, and prepare myself for dealing with pain. Many of my friends thought that visualizing pain was odd, but to set a 24-hour world record you experience a lot of pain. I worked on seeing myself ride through that pain, maintaining an aerodynamic position and staying on my race pace. When it was race day and I started to feel the effects of the intense Florida summer heat and humidity on my muscles, and the fatigue from pushing longer than I had in training, the pain was nothing compared to what I had visualized and prepared for. Many

months of visualization had prepared me to push way
beyond my imagined limits, and in my last world record I
rode 436 miles in 24 hours, actually breaking the tandem (a
bicycle built for two) record I had set nine months earlier.

Although some people don't want to think about the
pain or discomfort beforehand, for most people, visualization
can help cope with medical procedures like IV starts, bone
marrow biopsies, surgical pain, and other side effects of treatments. My patients who use visualization often need less pain
medication and tolerate their treatments better. They seem to
be more prepared and ready to cope with the challenges of
treatment. Many of my patients who are just starting the
Cancer Fitness exercise program set a personal goal and visualize themselves doing their activities in small steps that lead
up to achieving their goal. Some have set goals of climbing a
mountain and visualized climbing Mount Rainier and
within a year have done it! Others have aimed for the Danskin Triathlon, an Avon 3-day walk, or simply exercising regularly 3 days a week for 6 months.

The common denominator for the success of all my
patients is that they have all integrated visualization into their
life and exercise program and found success, but not without
the intensity, concentration, and enthusiasm that helped
them meet their goals. Your goals do not have to be competitive or highly athletic. Simply committing to a physically
active lifestyle may be a far greater and more challenging
goal to attain in the long term. Remembering to build in
small goals and rewards for your success can lead to a change
in your lifestyle.

Visualization extends beyond success in physical activity;
it can have positive effects on performing, giving a presentation, and coping with medical procedures. There is a large

body of research demonstrating the benefits of knowing what to expect about a medical procedure. From my experience, if you take that one more step and actually think about how you will cope and what you will look like during that time, the whole experience will be much less stressful and unpleasant.

In many ways, succeeding in exercise is a metaphor for succeeding in every aspect of life. Whether we are seeking to succeed in a regular exercise plan or another goal in life, carefully setting your goals, planning the steps to achieve them, and making the commitment to follow your plan is key to your success and accomplishment. This same formula will bring you success in anything you value and want to pursue.

THE LITTLE VOICES: SELF-TALK

The mental aspects of reaching your full potential cannot be separated from the physical. Your work and training must fit together in harmony. It takes time and discipline to develop and optimize the necessary skills to reach your highest potential, and your state of mind has a lot to do with eventual success in your pursuits. If you believe in yourself and your abilities and can see yourself accomplishing your goals, you will. Our self-dialogue has a way of becoming a self-fulfilling prophecy. Have you ever heard your mind say, "Don't trip on the sidewalk" and then whap, you trip. Your mind set you up to fall. I've had college students at graduation tell me they worried about falling up the stairs as they walked to get their diploma. They visualized falling and sure enough when it was their turn to walk up to the stage they tripped up the stairs. Turn off the negative voices, and visualize and listen to the positive voices. We are what we think, so think and visualize in a positive way.

Each of us is in a continual dialogue of thoughts running though our heads. As you become more aware of your self-talk, you may realize that while you are talking to a friend your mind is working on something else, or you are commenting to yourself about how beautiful the sunset is, what our schoolteachers used to call not paying attention. Recently I was giving a serious presentation to a group of powerful and somewhat intimidating scientists. I didn't think I was being particularly funny, but the audience certainly did. As I became more distracted and aware of their smiles and laughter, the little voices in my head started to wonder loudly and argue about just what it was that was so amusing. Was I giving the wrong talk? Did I have toilet paper on my shoe? Had I sat in something? I usually play to the audience when they are laughing, but the little voices were so terribly distracting that I tried to turn them off and make them go away by concentrating more on the slides and my talk. This time, the voices were remarkably persistent and vocal. However, my many years of training myself to stop the wicked little voices helped me to refocus my attention on the presentation, and eventually the little voices faded off into the background and went away. Regrettably, the smiles of my audience did not disappear with the voices and to this day I'm not sure what was so funny.

Our body and mind interact to effect a positive or negative outcome. How we see ourselves affects the way we interact with people. When we are threatened our mind talks to us. The little voices say "You can't do that," "You aren't good enough for that," or "You are too fat, thin, not smart enough." Our body physically responds to the self-talk in our mind and we aren't able to perform up to our potential, unless we train ourselves to turn off the negative voices and hear positive ones. Learning to stop the negative voices and reshape the negative thoughts into positive ones is a skill that takes practice and is key to achieving success in nonstressful and stressful situations.

When your little voices are talking to you, become aware of what you are saying. Listen to the words and the tone of the voices and learn to stop the negative and self-deprecating banter. When you feel good about yourself, what you are wearing, and what you are doing, you walk tall and feel confident. At these times, your voices are also giving you positive feedback. Many times the positive voices aren't as vocal as the negative ones and we don't realize the potential impact our positive self-talk could have on our daily life and actions. Tuning into the chatter in the back of your head and learning to stop the negative voices and reshape the negative thoughts into positive ones is key to achieving success.

MY GEOGRAPHY LESSON

My cycling began with a dream, a childhood dream that I think represented freedom, strength, and independence. Cycling is a pure sport that relies on a strong mind and body—and of course a reliable bicycle. The idea of riding from place to place, being efficient and coping with the natural elements, was freeing. When I first started cycling, I would ride around the neighborhood imagining what it would be like to ride across the United States; not over several months, but two or three weeks, training my body to be aerodynamic, making every pedal stroke count, and being efficient.

I was tipping the scales at the highest numbers I had ever seen; not my idea of being sleek or efficient. The idea of wearing tight lycra shorts that show every roll and dimple, even if they did have special padding for cycling, was out of the question—well, that is until I rode a few consecutive days in a row. Then I decided that perhaps black lycra would be acceptable. Doesn't black hide everything, almost?

I signed up for a cross-country tour, Pacific Atlantic Cycling Tour (PAC Tour), which was a 17-day transcontinental cross that was led by Susan Notorangelo and Lon Haldeman, two champions of distance cycling. They sent training instructions and stories of long climbs, big head winds, and fantastic adventure. I diligently started training, eventually getting to the point that I could ride 80 or 100 miles in the morning and then work an evening shift in the bone marrow transplant unit. When I reached that point of endurance, I started to feel confident. My next goal was to be able to do this cycling and working regimen two or three days in a row. I was getting strong and learning how to push though the fatigue and pain. Finally, the time came to begin the taper before the big event. I rested nearly 2 weeks and didn't work or stand on my legs much.

I boarded a United Airlines flight to San Diego and from my seat enjoyed the cloudless, clear mid-September day as we glided across the country. My window seat at the back of the plane afforded me an excellent view of the country's geography, which for some reason I had decided, before to this trip, was flat. As I sat there for hours looking at the endless folds and undulations and the vast, jagged mountain ranges, I started to seriously question my ability to ride across the U.S. in 17 days and wanted to cry. I thought northern Florida was "hilly." Why, Florida looked dead flat in the air compared to my airplane window view of Texas, Colorado, and California. My anxiety worsened as I was met in the San Diego airport by Lon and some of my cycling mates—lean men—and another woman who had far more cycling experience and visible muscle than me. Of course, fear interfered with any hope of sleeping that night as I envisioned being left in their dust or, even worse, lost in the desert.

The first day we rode only about 90 miles, climbing from the coast up to Julian, California. Driven by great fear of failure and humiliation, I struggled and wobbled steadily up to the summit of the climb. The next day was better, a big sescent in the dark and then fast roll through the desert. As the days went by I got stronger and more confident, but always had secret doubts about getting dropped and lost. The challenge of the PAC Tour taught me a lot about preparation, perseverance, and determination and about how important these qualities are, not only to following your dreams but also to success in achieving your dreams.

BALANCE: MIND/BODY INTEGRATION

When the mind and the body are in balance, everything seems to happen effortlessly and simply to flow. The concept of flow is not new. Mihaly Csikszentmihalyi, a professor of psychology at the University of Chicago, has written extensively about the idea. Although we strive to be in this harmonious balance, our mind and our body aren't always integrated as one. Distractions, anxiety, worry, and the daily chores and hassles of life often keep us from finding this balance and flow. Our previous discussion of the values of intensity, concentration, and enthusiasm are key components in finding this harmonious flow.

My mother is a horsewoman, and some days she describes her rides as "everything just clicked, DC [her somewhat neurotic horse] and I just moved together. It was like DC knew what I was thinking and I knew what he was thinking. We almost anticipated each other's moves." When everything works and Mom is one with her horse, she glows with happiness and the two of them seem to have a certain connectedness as they move effortlessly together. Other days, the mind/body balance isn't there and no matter how hard she and DC work, they don't quite reach that balance and flow.

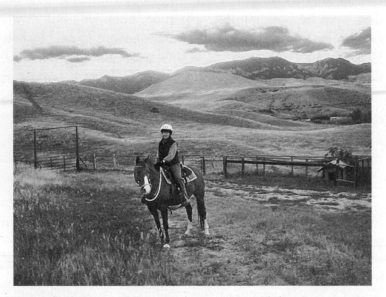

Christine working together as one with her horse.

The mind/body balance of flow doesn't occur just in physical activities. As I sit here writing tonight, the words are flowing easily. Yesterday, I sat and tried to force words, keenly aware of my anxiety about completing my work. When we watch a movie or read a book and get completely caught up in the story, we are in that balance or flow; completely present in the moment, absorbed and unaware of distractions in our mind or our surroundings. When this occurs, *intensity, concentration,* and *enthusiasm* are working together and we are in flow and can achieve a peak performance.

STOPPING

The hectic life of modern society is so rushed and frenetic that we seldom stop to enjoy the simple pleasures and beauty that surround us. Sometimes we need an event as shaking as cancer or another unforeseen, threatening incident to catch our attention enough to make us stop, perhaps long enough to reexamine our lives and listen to others and ourselves. Only by stopping can we develop the strength and courage to give our lives nothing but the best.

The diagnosis of cancer often causes one to feel the impermanence and fragility of life. How quickly and abruptly life can change and end—without warning and without logic. What has helped you survive previous life challenges, resist your disease, and fight on? For some it may be anger, or an intense love of life, or a wish to embrace life fully and be there for your children or grandchildren. We are all affected differently, but our emotional response can help us to see beyond the limitations of disease and understand the possibilities in our lives. Our hurried society does not look kindly on sitting idly and thinking about how things in our lives evolve and unfold. However, if we allow ourselves to stop and honestly evaluate our goals, ambitions, desires, and passions, we can muster the bravery and inner strength we need to look at new challenges and begin new adventures. It's through stopping and listening to our hearts that we can gather the energy and develop the grace and balance to reach beyond our dreams.

SEEING, BELIEVING, ACHIEVING

James was an insightful and sensitive 20-year-old man receiving a bone marrow transplant for non-Hodgkin's lymphoma. At the time he was diagnosed with lymphoma James had dropped out of school and was working two jobs he describes an "nonfulfilling." Now, in the sterile environment of the transplant unit, he felt isolated and as though his life was spinning out of control. At night, he would lie alone in his hospital room watching nothing but the flickering of the nightlight and listening to the endless steady clicking of his IV pump. He felt an incredible emptiness and loneliness and a certain isolation that serious illness can impart. Yet through this emotional turmoil, he could see himself thinking and moving in new directions. He said, "It was almost like I was floating on the ceiling looking down at myself and watching my ideals and values changing and becoming clearer. Maybe the drugs helped to intensify the experience? I don't know, but those endless nights were defining." James explained that he felt, "My new life was unfolding in the midst of the chaos of treatment, despite my uncertainty about the future. Suddenly, I developed a new passion and enthusiasm for life and a strong motivation and commitment to make a difference, not just survive. I saw that I could help other people. I wanted to do my best, beat this damned disease and try to make a difference for others." That was almost 13 years ago. Now James is Dr. James, a radiation oncologist taking care of cancer patients and offering hope and healing to all those he cares for.

SUMMARY

Bringing our lives into balance and pursuing interests and activities that we enjoy fosters intensity, concentration, and enthusiasm. The pursuit of excellence does not happen without commitment, passion, and a focused plan. Success does not happen by accident. Our dreams and our persistent struggle to make them real determine our future.

CLINICAL TRIALS RESEARCH: ADVANCING OUR UNDERSTANDING OF SCIENCE

There are so many decisions to be made when you are diagnosed with cancer, and one of the most important and time-sensitive considerations may be whether you want to participate in a clinical trials research study. Becoming involved in a clinical trials research study may offer you the best, cutting-edge treatment available at the time of your diagnosis, but there are decisions to make. This chapter will help you to have an understanding of what a clinical trials study is and what your rights are in making the decision to participate.

The studies that were reviewed in this book and form its scientific basis were all clinical trials. What we learned through these clinical trials has provided the basis for our current understanding of the benefits of exercise for cancer patients and survivors. Patients enrolled in these studies at various times during their treatment according to the *study protocol* (a set of rules used to run the study) were followed for different periods of time. From these studies we discovered that exercise can reduce the frequency and intensity of side effects and reduce risks for other long-term treatment-related side effects. All of the patients who enrolled in these studies had to weigh the risks and benefits of participating and decide if the study requirements and commitments were acceptable. These patients decided to participate for a variety of reasons but most often as a way to help their children and future generations, to improve their chances for survival, and to make a contribution to science and a difference to the world. Because of the generous spirit of these patients and their willingness to contribute their time and energy and true desire to make a contribution to this world, I am able to write this book and pass on what we have learned from our studies to, I hope, make a difference in your life.

WHAT IS A CLINICAL TRIAL?

Before a promising new experimental treatment for cancer or any other disease becomes standard therapy, research studies, known as clinical trials, are conducted to determine whether the new approach is both safe and effective. A clinical trial is started when a researcher or group of researchers believes that a certain new treatment or intervention may be of some value to the patient. Because researchers are seeking ways to prevent or cure a disease, such as cancer, or improve one's quality of life during or following cancer, there is an element of risk—the treatment may not cure or prevent the disease or even improve quality of life. However, without conducting the study we would not know whether a treatment or intervention is effective. We study how these interventions work and what the side effects may be, if and when they occur. Through these clinical studies we begin to learn the answers that lead to better treatments for cancer and ways to manage the side effects patients commonly experience from different types of treatments. Studies that are carefully conducted and well designed are the fastest and safest way to discover new effective treatments.

Participating in a clinical trial is an important decision faced by many cancer patients. You may be invited to participate in a clinical trial because your doctor thinks that the treatment may offer you the best chance of a cure, remission, or a better quality of life. When considering whether to participate, it is important for you to gather as much information about the study and ask as many questions as you may have. You want to be well informed and feel like you clearly understand what is involved in the study to be able to weigh the benefits and risks involved and whether participating in the study is right for you. Enrolling in a study is voluntary. Your health care team or the research team should explain the study to you and provide a copy of the consent form, which outlines the study procedures and potential risks and benefits. It is important to know that you can withdraw from the study at any time, even after you have signed the consent form and been enrolled in the study.

PHASES OF CLINICAL TRIALS

There are many different types of clinical trials. They include trials of cancer prevention, early detection, treatment, and quality of life. These studies are conducted in phases, especially studies that are examining new drugs or the use of an old drug for a new disease. The phases follow methodical steps:

- Phase 1. These are the earliest studies performed on humans to answer such questions as: How should a drug be given? How often should the drug be given? What is the optimal dose? Phase 1 trials study small groups of people, typically 20 to 80 participants, and focus on the safety of a drug or intervention, the dose range and determining what the side effects may be.
- Phase 2. These studies are conducted on larger groups of people, generally 110 to 300 participants, and focus on determining the effectiveness and continuing to examine the safety of the drug or intervention. Typical research questions are: What is the remission rate? What are the most common side effects? How does the intervention or drug reduce (or improve) a certain symptom, for example, pain or fatigue?
- Phase 3. At this phase of a clinical trial, the experimental treatment is looking promising and studies require larger groups of people, often as many as 1,000 or more. These studies address the question of how the experimental treatment compares to the usual treatment. Information continues to be collected to confirm the efficacy of the treatment and to monitor for side effects. Results from phase 3 studies provide information that allows the drug or treatment to be used safely and commercially.
- Phase 4. These studies are also called aftermarket

studies, because the drug or intervention is commercially available. Phase 4 trials continue to test the product (drug or treatment) to determine its effectiveness in different populations and also to determine if there are any side effects with regular long-term use.

PARTICIPATING IN A TRIAL

All clinical trials follow a protocol that has specific guidelines about who qualifies to participate. These guidelines are based on such factors as age, gender, type and stage of disease, medical history, and current medical condition. You qualify for a clinical trial if you meet the specific guidelines of the protocol, also called the inclusion and exclusion criteria. These criteria are not used to reject people but rather to identify the individuals who might benefit the most from the trial, maintain safety, and ensure that the research question can be answered.

For example, many times patients have asked to participate in one of my exercise studies because they like to exercise or they think it may help them with their treatment. Upon further questioning, they may not be eligible to enroll in the study because of prior illnesses or the type of chemotherapy they are receiving or simply because they exercise too much. Determining eligibility is important for the protection of the research participants and the integrity of a study.

WHAT HAPPENS IN A TRIAL

If you are invited to participate in a study you will be given information about the study and the procedures that are required. You will be given a consent form that gives specific information about the study, who is eligible, why the study is being conducted, and your risks and benefits. Be sure you have taken the time to read the form, have adequate time to think about the study, and have asked all of your questions. Understanding what is involved in the study and the study expectations, risks, and benefits is important and all part of the informed consent process. The informed consent process is very important and is a way to insure that your rights and safety are protected. Before a study can begin recruiting and enrolling patients, an institutional review board (IRB) must approve the study and consent form. The IRB consists of a group of professionals and lay people who examine the study protocol and all the study materials to determine if the study is safe and ethical and does not create any undue or unnecessary risk to the patient.

Some studies require more tests and doctor visits than you might normally have for the treatment of your illness. The research team will keep you informed of follow-up appointments. Following the protocol, or study guidelines, is important for your safety and the ultimate success of the study. Stay in close contact with the research team, and don't be afraid to ask questions during the study.

Study designs vary. Some use a placebo, which is an inactive pill, liquid, or powder that has no therapeutic value. Placebo trials are used to compare the effectiveness of another treatment. Other studies may be blinded, or masked. A blinded study may be single blind, in which case participants do not know whether they are in the experimental or control group, or double blind, in which case neither the study staff nor the participants know who is receiving the experimental treatment. A double-blind design is used so that neither the doctor's nor the patient's expectations about the experiment will influence the outcome.

RISKS AND BENEFITS

There are risks and benefits to everything we choose to do in life, and research is no exception. Participating in a clinical trial offers several benefits: (1) you are taking an active role in your health care, (2) you have access to state-of-the-art treatment that is not yet available to everyone with your condition, (3) you may obtain medical care by leading medical experts while you are in the trial, and (4) you are making a contribution to medical research, to society, and to those who follow.

The risks of participating in a clinical trial should be understood before you consent to participate. These risks may include (1) experiencing side effects of the medications or treatment that are specific to the study, (2) realizing that the treatment may not work for you, and (3) giving a lot of your time to participate and adhere to the protocol, which may mean additional trips to the study site, extra tests, complicated drug or treatment regimens, or keeping a log.

When you read the informed consent and discuss the study with your doctor or the research team, ask questions so that you understand the risks and benefits of the study. You have to make the decision to participate, and without a clear understanding of the risks and benefits, it's difficult to make an informed and educated decision. Remember, though, you can always stop participating in the study if you enroll and then later decide you really don't want to participate.

QUALITY-OF-LIFE RESEARCH

Lou was a 67-year-old rancher recently diagnosed with lung cancer. He was feeling downhearted and depressed by what he saw as a glum and grim future, and wondered how he would be able to oversee the ranch and family business. He was still recovering from surgery and not feeling strong or capable of doing most of his usual activities, and the idea of starting chemotherapy before he felt better filled him with dread. Lou and his family traveled over five hours to the cancer center where he was receiving treatment. During his last visit, Lou's doctor had given him some information about the standard treatment for his form of lung cancer and information about a clinical trial research study he was eligible to participate in. Lou discussed his treatment options at great length with his family. They weighed the pros and cons and came to the conclusion that because of the great distance they traveled to get to the cancer center for treatment, the clinical trial would be too much of a burden. Lou met with his oncologist to discuss his decision to follow the standard treatment but said that if there were other studies that didn't require so much time and travel he would be interested in participating. Lou's doctor told him about our exercise studies. Lou did not know that there were studies about how to improve one's quality of life. When he learned that the study didn't require any additional travel and that he could perform the exercises at home, he was delighted to qualify and be enrolled. Lou said, "The exercise study complemented my care, and I felt like I was not only doing something for myself, but maybe helping other people learn to live a better life with cancer. The exercise seemed to improve my mood and make me feel more hopeful about life and getting through this darn treatment."

QUESTIONS TO ASK BEFORE DECIDING TO PARTICIPATE

Prepare for your meeting with the research team in advance. If you have the informed consent, read it before your meeting and write down your questions. Bring a friend or family member with you to ask questions and be another set of ears to hear the answers to your questions. It may also be helpful to bring a tape recorder so you can replay the discussion, or a notepad so you can later review your notes about the discussion.

Following are some questions that may help you in making your decisions about participating in a clinical trial. Use these questions to start your own list of questions that are specific to your situation and the study you are considering:

What other treatment options do I have?
Why is the study being done? By whom?
Who is sponsoring the study?
Why do you think I will benefit from the study?
What treatments or extra tests will I have during the study?
How long will I be in the study?

Are there medicines or activities I should avoid while in the study?

What are the risks of the study compared with approved treatments?

Are there any long-term risks or side effects?

What are the costs? Who pays for the study? Will insurance cover my expenses?

What are my rights as a study subject?

How are my privacy and confidentiality and medical records protected?

The Experience of Being in a Study

Debbie was a 36-year-old librarian when she was diagnosed with an aggressive form of breast cancer. At the time of diagnosis she felt overwhelmed by emotion and all the decisions that needed to be made. When Debbie met with her medical oncologist for the initial consultation and discussion about treatment options, she was given three different chemotherapy choices. One of her choices was to be in a clinical trials research study. The study offered Debbie cutting-edge treatment and the opportunity to get the best care available; the down side was that the treatment regimen was more aggressive, which meant she got chemotherapy more often and might experience worse side effects. Debbie and her husband, Matt, listened to the doctor, took notes about her treatment options, and took the consent form for the study home to review. At home, Debbie and Matt talked about the risks and benefits of each of the treatment options and the chances for a cure. Even though the research study required more time at the cancer center, and additional tests (which were all paid for by the study), she decided to enroll in the study. Debbie wanted to have the best chance for a cure and to give back whatever she could to science and the world. Debbie describes her feelings about participating in the study as, "I feel like I not only got the best medicine available at the time of my diagnosis, but that I was able to offer something to science, help other women with this disease, and being in the study just made me feel like I was able to do something good for the world. I've been cancer-free for four years, and looking back I wouldn't have changed my decision. The treatment was hard, but I think any kind of chemotherapy isn't much fun, and I'm thankful that I was given the opportunity to make a difference and a contribution."

HOW DO I FIND OUT ABOUT CLINICAL TRIALS IN MY AREA?

Often the best way to learn about clinical trials research programs that you may be eligible for is to ask your health care team. They may be conducting studies for which you qualify. The web is also a good place to learn about clinical trials being conducted in your area or that are open to enrollment that you may be interested in participating in. Some websites that may be helpful are listed here:

- These sites provide general information about clinical trials.
    www.ClinicalTrials.gov
    www.CenterWatch.com
- These sites provide information about specific tri-

als that are open and funded by the National Institutes of Health.

  www.cc.nih.gov index.cgi

  clinicalstudies.info.nih.gov

- This site provides information about the federal
  codes relating to the protection of human subjects'
  rights:

  ohrp.osophs.dhhs.gov/humansubjects guidance
    45cfr46

- The Coalition of National Cancer Cooperative
  Groups hosts a website called TrialCheck, which
  provides access to physicians and other health care
  professions about cancer clinical trials information.
  The TrialCheck search engine queries a database
  of approximately 400 Cooperative Group cancer
  clinical trials that are open and enrolling eligible
  patients. A Cooperative Group is a group of medical oncologists or radiation oncologists who work
  together to conduct large clinical trials in an effort
  to get studies done quickly, efficiently, and with
  the scientific rigor necessary to change standards
  of treatment and care of cancer patients. Some of
  the oncology groups are: Radiation Therapy
  Oncology Group (RTOG), Eastern Cooperative
  Oncology Group (ECOG), Cancer and Leukemia
  Group B (CALGB), National Surgical Adjuvant
  Breast and Bowel Project (NSABP), and South-
  west Oncology Group (SWOG).

  www.trialcheck.org

- HopeLink Clinical Trial Service is a free and con-
  fidential service provided by the Oncology Nursing Society. HopeLink provides assistance in

locating a clinical trial that meets your personal needs. This service can help you determine if you meet preliminary eligibility requirements for select trials and then permits you to submit your information online to the organizations conducting the trial.

www.hopelink.com clinicaltrials

SUMMARY

Participating in a clinical trials research study may increase your chances of an optimal outcome because you will be receiving the best treatment available and gives you the opportunity to make a difference for science and humanity. However, you must consider the risks of participating, which may mean unusual side effects from a new drug and extra time spent getting medical tests or for doctor visits. Our understanding of science and how to treat cancer is improved through clinical trials research and all the patients who participated in the trials. The exercise research presented in this book was made available in part by research grants, but mostly because of the patients who were willing to step out and take a risk to see if exercise would make a difference. We've learned a lot through all of the study participants, and now I am able to pass this knowledge on to you.

CANCER FITNESS CONTRACT

I,——————, have agreed to dutifully follow the Cancer Fitness exercise program for 12 weeks. I will begin by making a complete list of the reasons I want to start this program and all the possible barriers and excuses that I think I might encounter along the way. I will strive to make reasonable and achievable weekly goals and keep a record of my exercise accomplishments in an exercise log. I know that if I set unreasonable goals I will not succeed but that I can revise my goals to make them realistic. I willingly acknowledge that there may be obstacles to my progress that may present a challenge that may necessitate revising my goals but that these challenges will not prevent me from completing the program.

I sign this contract today with my friend and/or exercise companion, who is my witness.

_____

Signed

_____

Date

_____

Printed Name

_____

Friend/Exercise Companion/Witness

RESISTANCE EXERCISE LOGS

RESISTANCE EXERCISE A

Exercises	Date			Date			Date	
	Reps+Sets	Band Color/Wt		Reps+Sets	Band Color/Wt		Reps+Sets	Band Color/Wt
Squats								
Lat pull-downs								
Leg extension								
Flies								
Hip adduction								
Bicep curls								
Hip abduction								

RESISTANCE EXERCISE B

Exercises	Date			Date			Date	
	Reps+Sets	Band Color/Wt		Reps+Sets	Band Color/Wt		Reps+Sets	Band Color/Wt
Lunges								
Bench Press								
Hamstring Curls								
Bent Rows								
Hip Extension								
Bicep curls								
Tricep Extension								
Crucnhes								

AEROBIC EXERCISE LOG

Date: **Time:**   **Weather:**

Place:

Activity:

Time:

RPE:

Grade:

Date: **Time:**   **Weather:**

Place:

Activity:

Time:

RPE:

Grade:

Date: **Time:**   **Weather:**

Place:

Activity:

Time:

RPE:

Grade:

OTHER RESOURCES
FOR SUPPORT AND INFORMATION

General Resources

American Cancer Society
www.cancer.org
800-ACS-2345

Cancer Resources
457 West 22nd Street, Suite B
New York, NY 10011
Phone: 800-401-2233
Fax: 212-243-1063
www.cancerresources.com

CancerSource.com
400-1 Totten Pond Road
Waltham, MA 02451-2051
www.cancersource.com

Centers for Disease Control
www.cdc.gov/cancer/prostate:
This site provides information about cancer prevention in
general and specifically related to a variety of different types
of cancers.

Lance Armstrong Foundation
P.O. Box 161150
Austin, TX 78716-1150
Phone: 512-236-8820
Fax: 512-236-8482
www.laf.org

National Cancer Institute, National Institutes of Health
Cancer Information Service (CIS)
Phone: 800-4-CANCER (800-422-6237)
cis.nci.nih.gov: Information about all forms of cancer and treatment.
www.nci.nih.gov/clinical_trials/understanding: Information about clinical trials that may be open for patients with different types and stages of cancer.

National Coalition for Cancer Survivorship
1010 Wayne Avenue, Suite 770
Silver Spring, MD 20910
Telephone: 301-650-9127 or 877-622-7937
Fax: 301-565-9670
www.cansearch.org
www.cancerindex.org: Excellent site to obtain general information and direction about where to go for more detailed information regarding specific cancers and blood disorders.

National Lymphedema Network
800-541-3259
www.lymphnet.org

Association of Cancer Online Resources
www.acor.org

Breast Cancer

National Alliance of Breast Cancer Organizations
9 East 37th Street, 10th Floor
New York, NY 10016
www.nabco.org

Y-ME National Breast Cancer Organization
212 W.Van Buren, Suite 500
Chicago, IL 60607
Phone: 312-986-8338
Fax: 312-294-8597
www.y-me.org

Susan G. Komen Foundation
P. O. Box 650309
Dallas, TX 75265-0309.
Phone: 800-I-MAWARE
(800-462-9273)
www.komen.org

National Breast Cancer Coalition
1707 L Street, NW, Suite 1060
Washington, DC 20036
Phone: 202-296-7477
Fax: 202-265-6854
www.natlbcc.org

The Breast Cancer Fund
2107 O'Farrell Street
San Francisco, CA 94115
Phone: 415-346-8223

Fax: 415-346-2975
www.breastcancerfund.org/about.htm

The Breast Cancer Research Foundation
654 Madison Avenue, Suite 1209
New York, NY 10021
Phone: 646-497-2600
www.bcrfcure.org

Team Survivor
1223 Wilshire Blvd. #570
Santa Monica, CA 90403
www.teamsurvivor.org/contact/index.html

Bone Cancer and Sarcoma

Bone Cancer International, Inc.
P.O. Box 504
Newbury Park, CA 91319-0504
Phone: 805-480-3551
Fax: 805-375-1946.
www.bonecancer.to toc.html

Sarcoma Alliance
775 East Blithedale, #334
Mill Valley, CA 94941
Phone: 415-381-7236
www.sarcomaalliance.com

Sarcoma Foundation of America
P.O. Box 458

Damascus, MD 20872
www.curesarcoma.org

Carcinoma

The Carcinoid Cancer Foundation, Inc.
333 Mamaroneck Avenue #492
White Plains, NY 10605
Phone:888-722-3132 or 914-683-1001
www.carcinoid.org

Colon Cancer

Colon Cancer Alliance, Inc.
175 Ninth Avenue
New York, NY 10011
Phone: 212-627-7451
Toll free: 877-422-2030
Fax: 425-940-6147
www.ccalliance.org

Kidney Cancer

National Kidney Cancer Association
1234 Sherman Ave., Suite 203
Evanston, IL 60202
Phone: 800-850-9132 toll-free
www.nkca.org

Leukemia and Lymphoma

The Lymphoma Research Foundation
8800 Venice Blvd., Suite 207
Los Angeles, CA
Phone: 310-204-7040
Helpline: 800-500-9976
www.lymphoma.org

The Leukemia & Lymphoma Society
1311 Mamaroneck Avenue
White Plains, NY 10605
Phone: 914-949-5213
Fax: 914-949-6691
www.leukemia.org/hm_lls

Leukemia Research Foundation
820 Davis Street, Suite 420
Evanston, IL 60201
Phone: 847-424-0600
Fax: 847-424-0606
www.leukemia-research.org/contact.asp

Chronic Lymphocytic Leukemia Foundation
1415 Louisiana, Suite 3625
Houston, TX 77002
Phone: 713-752-2350
www.cllfoundation.org

Mycosis Fungoides Foundation
PO Box 374
Birmingham, MI 48102–0374
Phone: 248–644–9014

Liver Cancer

Allegheny General Liver Cancer Program
320 East North Avenue
Pittsburgh, PA 15212-4772
Phone: 412–359–6738
Fax: 412–359–6288
www.livercancer.com

Lung Cancer

Alliance for Lung Cancer
500 W. 8th St., Suite 240
Vancouver, WA 98660
Lung Cancer Hotline: 800–298–2436 (U.S. only)
Phone: 360–696–2436
Fax: 360 735-1305
www.alcase.org

The American Lung Association
61 Broadway, 6th Floor
New York, NY 10006
212-315-8700
www.lungusa.org

Lung Cancer Toll-Free
information line for lung cancer support:
877-646-LUNG (877-646-5864)
www.lungcancer.org

Myeloma Foundation

International Myeloma Foundation
12650 Riverside Drive, Suite 206
North Hollywood, CA 91607-3421
Toll Free: 800-452-2873 (U.S. and Canada)
Phone: 818-487-7455 (elsewhere)
Fax: 818-487-7454
mffoundation.org
www.myeloma.org/myeloma/home.jsp

Ovarian Cancer

Gilda's Club Worldwide
322 Eighth Avenue, Suite 1402
New York, NY 10001
www.gildasclub.org/contactus

National Ovarian Cancer Coalition, Inc.
500 NE Spanish River Boulevard, Suite 14
Boca Raton, FL 33431
Toll free: 888-OVARIAN
Phone: 561-393-0005
Fax: 561-393-7275
www.ovarian.org

Pancreatic Cancer

Pancreatica.org
5 Harris Court

Building N, Suite 3
Monterey, California 93940
Phone: 831-658-0600
www.pancreatica.org

Prostate Cancer

National Prostate Cancer Coalition
1154 15th St., NW
Washington, DC 20005
Phone: 202-463-9455
Toll-free: 888-245-9455
Fax: 202-463-9456
www.4npcc.org

Prostate Cancer Research Institute
5777 W. Century Blvd, Suite 885
Los Angeles, CA 90045
Phone: 310-743-2110
Fax: 310-743-2113
www.prostate-cancer.org

Prostate Cancer Research Foundation of Canada
1262 Don Mills Road, Suite 1-F
Toronto, ON M3B 2W7
Canada
Phone: 416-441-2131
Toll-free: 888-255-0333
Fax: 416-441-2325
www.prostatecancer.on.ca

Prostate Cancer Support Groups
5003 Fairview Avenue
Downers Grove, IL 60515
Phone: 630-795-1002
Fax: 630-795-1602
PCa Support Hotline: 800-80-US TOO
(800-808-7866)
www.ustoo.com

Skin Cancer

American Melanoma Foundation
3914 Murphy Canyon Road, Suite A132
San Diego, CA 92123
Phone: 858-277-4426
www.melanomafoundaton.org

The Melanoma Research Foundation
23704-5 El Toro Rd. #206
Lake Forest, CA 92630
800-MRF-1290
www.melanoma.org

Testicular Cancer

Lance Armstrong Foundation (see General Resources, p.246)

Thyroid Cancer

Thyroid Cancer Survivors' Association, Inc.
PO Box 1545
New York, NY 10159–1545
Phone: 877-588-7904 (toll free)
Fax: 630-604-6078
www.thyca.org

Professional Organizations

Association of Oncology Social Workers
1211 Locust Street
Philadelphia, PA 19107
Phone: 215-599-6093
Fax: 215 545 8107
www.aosw.org

American Society of Clinical Oncology

People Living with Cancer
American Society of Clinical Oncology
1900 Duke Street, Suite 200
Alexandria, VA 22314
Phone: 703-797-1914
Fax: 703-299-1044
www.peoplelivingwithcancer.org

Oncology Nursing Society
125 Enterprise Drive
Pittsburgh, PA 15275
Phone: 866-257-4ONS (toll free)
Fax: 877-369-5497 (toll free)
www.ons.org

Other Helpful Websites

www.oncolink.com
www.meds.com/cancerlinks: Provides direct links to other
cancer resource sites on the web.

GLOSSARY

Aerobic exercise. Continuous and sustained exercise that increases your heart rate.

Antiemetic. A medication to prevent or reduce nausea and vomiting.

Bone mass. The total amount of bone in the body.

Bone mineral density (BMD) or bone density. The amount of mineralized bone in one's body.

Chemotherapy. Drugs used to treat a disease, in this case cancer; can be given by mouth or by vein.

Clinical trial. A research study in which participants are randomly assigned to treatment group(s); the treatment may be medication, diet, exercise.

Dual-energy x-ray absorptiometry (DXA or DEXA). A common and accurate test to measure bone density in the body and at specific sites, such as the hip or spine.

Epidemiology. The science of the cause and spread of disease.

Functional ability. How much and how easily one is able to complete tasks; influenced by muscle strength and heart and lung fitness.

Immunotherapy. Treatment that increases the body's natural defense system to control or remove cancer cells.

Lymphedema. Swelling in an arm or leg from the removal of lymph nodes or from radiation therapy.

Macrocycle. The accumulation of mesocydes.

Malignancy. A cancerous growth with the ability to grow and spread.

Menopause. Cessation of menstruation. Occurs naturally between the ages of 45 and 55. Early menopause can be cause by some forms of chemotherapy or by surgery that removes the ovaries (oophorectomy).

Mesocycle. Three or four weeks of exercise broken into periods of higher and lower intensity exercise.

Metastasis. The spread of cancer cells to distant parts of the body through the blood or lymphatic systems.

Microcycle. Exercise done in 7 days or for over 1 week.

Mucositis. Redness and sores in the mouth that occur with some chemotherapy treatments.

Osteopenia. Low bone density that is between 1 and 2.5 standard deviations below the mean for young normal adults.

Osteoporosis. Low bone mass and density that is less than 2.5 standard deviations below the mean for young normal adults; a chronic progressive condition that can lead to bone fractures.

Peripheral neuropathy. A reduction or complete loss of sensation occurring most frequently in the fingers and toes, caused by some chemotherapy drugs.

Placebo. An inert pill, liquid, or powder that has no therapeutic value.

Protocol. A set of rules used in a study to ensure that the right participants are enrolled and the study procedures are adhered to.

Radiation therapy. A cancer treatment using high-energy X-ray beams.

Rating of perceived exertion (RPE). A way to determine or rate how hard you are exercising.

Recurrence. A return of cancer in the same location or another site.

Remission. Complete or partial disappearance of detectable or measurable disease.

Repetitions. The number of times you move a weight though one complete exercise.

Resistance exercise. Exercises such as weight lifting or using a band to pull or push against a force to increase muscle strength.

Sets. Number of times you do an exercise, rest, and then return to do the exercise again (e.g., 8 repetitions of leg extensions done 3 times, or 3 sets)

Strength training. See **Resistance exercise.**

Usual care. Standard of care for a particular illness; one who is not receiving the experimental treatment.

Weight-bearing exercise. Exercises that require the legs to support the body, such as walking or running.

SUGGESTED READING

Following are some of the references I used in compiling the information for this book. Some of these articles can be found on the web, and others can be obtained through a medical library.

Blanchard CM, Courneya KS, Rodgers WM, and Murnaghan DM. Determinants of exercise intention and behavior in survivors of breast and prostate cancer: an application of the theory of planned behavior. *Cancer Nursing.* Apr;25(2):88–95, 2002.

Byers T, Nestle M, McTiernan A, Doyle C, Currie-Williams A, Gansler T, and Thun M. American Cancer Society guidelines on nutrition and physical activity for cancer prevention: reducing the risk of cancer with healthy food choices and physical activity. *CA Cancer Journal for Clinicians.* Mar–Apr;52(2):92–119, 2002.

Chlebowski RT, Aiello E, and McTiernan A. Weight loss in breast cancer patient management. *Journal of Clinical Oncology.* Feb 15;20(4):1128–1143, Review, 2002.

Courneya KS, Blanchard CM, and Lang, DM. Exercise adherence in breast cancer survivors training for a dragon boat race competition: a preliminary investigation. *Psychooncology.* Sep–Oct;10(5):444-4-52, 2001.

Courneya KS, and Freidenreich CM. Relationship between exercise pattern across the cancer experience and current quality of life in colorectal cancer survivors. *Journal of Alternative and Complementary Medicine*. Fall;3(3):215–26, 1997.

Demark-Wahnefried W, Hars V, Conaway MR, Havlin K, Rimer BK, McElveen G, and Winer EP. Reduced rates of metabolism and decreased physical activity in breast cancer patients receiving adjuvant chemotherapy. *American Journal of Clinical Nutrition*. 65:1495, 1997.

Dimeo FC, Fetscher S, Lange W, Mertelsmann R, and Keul J. Effects of aerobic exercise on the physical performance and incidence of treatment-related complications after high-dose chemotherapy. *Blood,* 90:3390–3394, 1997.

Dimeo FC, Rumberger BG, and Keul J. Aerobic exercise as therapy for cancer fatigue. *Medicine and Science in Sports and Exercise*. 30(4): 475–478, 1998.

Dimeo FC, Stieglitz RD, Novelli-Fischer U, Fetscher S, Mertelsmann R, and Keul J. Correlations between physical performance and fatigue in cancer patients. *Annals of Oncology,* 8: 1251–1255, 1997.

Dimeo FC, Stieglitz RD, Novelli-Fischer U, Fetscher S, and Keul, J. Effects of physical activity on the fatigue and psychologic status of cancer patients during chemotherapy. *Cancer,* 85(10): 2273–2277, 1999.

Dimeo FC, Tilmann MHM, Bertz H, Kanz L, Mertelsmann R, and Keul J. Aerobic exercise in the rehabilitation of cancer patients after high-dose chemotherapy and autologous stem cell transplantation. *Cancer*. 79:1717–1722, 1997.

Dishman RK. Determinants of participation in physical activity. In Bouchard C, Shepard RJ, Stephens T, et al. (eds.) *Exercise, Fitness and Health*. Champaign IL: Human Kinetics Books, 1998, pp. 75–101.

Evenson KR, Wilcox S, Pettinger M, Brunner R, King AC, and McTiernan A. Vigorous leisure activity through women's adult life: the Women's Health Initiative Observational Cohort Study. *American Journal of Epidemiology.* Nov; 15;156(10):945–953, 2002.

Fairey AS, Courneya KS, Field CJ, Mackey JR. Physical exercise and immune system function in cancer survivors: a comprehensive review and future directions. *Cancer.* Jan 15;94(2):539–551, Review, 2002.

Godfrey, CM. "Yes" to exercise for breast cancer survivors. *Canadian Medical Association Journal.* Dec1;159(11):1358, 1998.

Hovi L, Era P, Rautonen J, and Siimes MA. Impaired muscle strength in female adolescents and young adults surviving leukemia in childhood. *Cancer.* Jul 1;72(1):276–281, 1993.

Jenney M, Faragher B, Jones P, and Woodcock A. Lung function and exercise capacity in survivors of childhood leukemia. *Medical and Pediatric Oncology.* 24:222–230, 1995.

Jones LW, and Courney KS Exercise discussions during cancer treatment consultations. *Cancer Practice.* Mar–Apr;10(2): 66–74, 2002.

Keats MR, Courneya KS, Danielsen S., and Whitsett SF Leisure-time physical activity and psychosocial well-being in adolescents after cancer diagnosis. *Journal of Pediatric Oncology.* 16:180–188, 1999.

Kent H. Breast-cancer survivors begin the challenge to exercise taboos. *Canadian Medical Association Journal.* Oct 1;55(7):969–971, 1996.

Kohl HW. Physical activity and cardiovascular disease: evidence for a dose response. *Medicine and Science in Sports and Exercise.* Jun:33(6Suppl):S472–483, 2001.

Layne J, and Nelson M. The effects of progressive resistance training on bone density: a review. *Medicine and Science in Sports and Exercise.* 31(1):25-30, 1999.

Lee IM, and Skerrett PJ. Physical activity and all-cause mortality: what is the dose response relation? *Medicine and Science in Sports and Exercise.* Jun:33(6Suppl):S459–471, 2001.

MacVicar MG, and Winningham ML. Promoting the functional capacity of cancer patients. *Cancer Bulletin,* 38:235–239, 1986.

Maguire GP, Lee EG, Bevington DJ, Kuchemann CS, Crabtree RJ, and Cornell C. Psychiatric problems in the first year after mastectomy. *British Medical Journal.* 1:963–967, 1978.

Martinsen EW. The role of aerobic exercise in the treatment of depression. *Stress Medicine,* 3:93–100, 1987.

Matthys D, Verhaaren H, Benoiit Y, Laureys G, De Naeyer A, and Craen M. Gender differences in aerobic capacity in adolescents after cure from malignant disease in childhood. *Acta Paediatrica.* 82:459–462, 1993.

McTiernan A. Physical activity and the prevention of breast cancer. *Medscape Womens Health.* Sep–Oct;5(5):E1, Review, 2000.

McTiernan A, Ulrich C, Kumai C, Schwartz R, Mahloch J, Hastings R, Gralow J, and Potter JD. Anthropometric and hormone effects of an eight-week exercise-diet intervention in breast cancer patients; results of a pilot study. *Cancer, Epidemiology, Biomarkers and Prevention.* 7:477–481, 1998.

Mock V, Burke MB, Sheehan P, Creaton EM, Winningham ML, McKenney-Tedder S, Schwager LP, and Liebman M. A nursing rehabilitation program for women with breast cancer receiving adjuvant chemotherapy. *Oncology Nursing Forum.* 21:899–907, 1994.

Mock V, Dow KH, Meares CJ, Grimm PM, Dienemann JA, Haisfield-Wolfe ME, Quitasol W, Mitchell S, Chakravarthy A, and Gage I. An exercise intervention for management of fatigue and emotional distress during radiotherapy treatment for breast cancer. *Oncology Nursing Forum.* 24:991–1000, 1997.

Morgan, WP. Anxiety reduction following acute physical activity. *Psychiatric Annals.* 9: 36–45, 1979.

Moses J, Steptoe A, Mathews A, and Edwards S. The effects of exercise training on mental well-being in the normal populations: a controlled trial. *Journal of Psychosomatic Research.* 33: 47–61, 1989.

Pinto BM, and Maruyama NC. Exercise in the rehabilitation of breast cancer survivors. *Psychooncology* May–June;8(3): 191–206, 1999.

Polinsky M. Functional status of long-term breast cancer survivors: demonstrating chronicity. *Health and Social Work.* 3: 166–77, 1994.

Rockhill B, Willett WC, Manson JE, Leitzmann MF, Stampfer MJ, Hunter DJ, and Colditz GA. Physical activity and mortality: a prospective study among women. *American Journal of Public Health.* 91(4):578–583, 2001.

Rose MA. Health promotion and risk prevention: applications for cancer survivors. *Oncology Nursing Forum.* May–June;16(3):335–340, 1998.

Roth DL, and Holmes DS. Influences of aerobic exercise training in and relaxation training on physical and psychologic health following stressful life events. *Psychosomatic Medicine,* 49:355–365, 1987.

Schwartz AL. Fatigue mediates the effects of exercise on quality of life in women with breast cancer. *Quality of Life Research.* 8:529–538, 1999.

Schwartz, AL. Weight change in women who do and do not exercise during adjuvant chemotherapy for breast cancer. *Cancer Practice*, 8:229–237, 2000a.

Schwartz AL. Daily fatigue patterns and effects of exercise in women with breast cancer. *Cancer Practice*, 8(1):16–24, 2000b.

Schwartz AL. *Cancer.* In Moore G (ed.) *Exercise Prescription in Chronic Disease.* Champaign, IL: Human Kinetics Books, 2001, pp. 252–267.

Schwartz AL. Effects of exercise on bone density and body composition of breast cancer patients receiving chemotherapy. *Medicine and Science in Sports Exercise.* 33(S276, 1557) 2002a.

Schwartz AL. Effects of exercise on bone mineral density in pre-and postmenopausal women receiving chemotherapy for breast cancer. *Journal of Clinical Oncology.* 21(Part 1, 1416), 2002b.

Schwartz AL, King M, Samson C, and Holub J. A randomized trial of exercise for newly diagnosed patients receiving chemotherapy: effects on bone density and body composition. *Oncology Nursing Forum.* 29(336 20), 2002.

Schwartz AL, Mori M, Gao R, Nail LM, and King ME. Exercise reduces daily fatigue in women with breast cancer receiving chemotherapy. *Medicine and Science in Sports and Exercise.* 33:718–723, 2001.

Schwartz AL, Thompson JT, Masood N. Interferon induced fatigue in melanoma: a pilot study of exercise and methylphenidate. *Oncology Nursing Forum* 29(7 web feature), 2002.

Segar ML, Katch, VL, Roth RS, Garcia AW, Portner TI, Glickman SG, Haslanger S, and Wilkins EG. The effect of aerobic exercise on self-esteem and depressive and anxiety symptoms among breast cancer survivors. *Oncology Nursing Forum.* Jan–Feb;25(1):107–113, 1998.

Sharkey A, Carey AB, Heise CT, and Barber G. Cardiac rehabilitation after cancer therapy in children and young adults. *American Journal of Cardiology.* 71:1488–1490, 1993.

Shors AR, Solomon C, McTiernan A, and White E. Melanoma risk in relation to height, weight, and exercise. *Cancer Causes Control.* Sep;12(7):599–606, 2001.

Stone P, Richardson A, Ream E, Smith AG, Kerr DJ, and Kearney N. Cancer-related fatigue: inevitable, unimportant and untreatable. Results of a multi-centre patient survey. *Annals of Oncology.* 11:971–997, 2000.

Tworoger SS, Yasui Y, Ulrich CM, Nakamura H, LaCroix K, Johnston R, and McTiernan A. Mailing strategies and recruitment into an intervention trial of the exercise effect on breast cancer biomarkers. *Cancer Epidemiology Biomarkers and Prevention.* Jan;11(1):73–77, 2002.

Warner JT, Bell W, Webb GK, and Gregory JW. Daily energy expenditure and physical activity in survivors of childhood malignancy. *Pediatric Research.* May:43(5):607–613, 1998.

Wyatt G, and Friedman LL. Long-term female cancer survivors: quality of life issues and clinical implications. *Cancer Nursing.* Feb;19(1):1–7, 1996.

Young-McCaughan S, and Sexton DL. A retrospective investigation of the relationship between aerobic exercise and quality of life in women with breast cancer. *Oncology Nursing Forum.* 18:751–757, 1991.

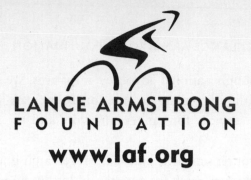

LANCE ARMSTRONG
F O U N D A T I O N
www.laf.org

The Lance Armstrong Foundation (LAF) exists to enhance the quality of life for those living with, through, and beyond cancer. We want to continue to define, refine, and improve cancer survivor resources and facilitate the delivery of services—and a large dose of hope—to the patients, their families, and other loved ones touched by the disease. It's a tall order, but an organization that bears the name of the man who came back from cancer to win four consecutive Tour de France victories can aim for nothing less.

Founded in 1997 by cancer survivor and champion cyclist Lance Armstrong, the LAF's mission is to enhance the quality of survival of those diagnosed with cancer. We seek to promote the optimal physical, psychological, and social recovery and care of cancer survivors and their loved ones. The LAF focuses its activities in the following areas: survivorship education and resources, community programs, national advocacy initiatives, and scientific and clinical research grants.

- Through survivorship education and resources, we educate cancer survivors, health care professionals, and the general public about cancer survivorship issues.
- Through innovative community programs, we aid in the development of after-treatment services and support for survivors.

- Through national advocacy initiatives, we address health policy issues in an effort to increase support and services for cancer survivors and their loved ones.
- Through scientific and clinical research grants, we support research for a better understanding of cancer and cancer survivorship.

Providing information, services, and support, the LAF strives to help all cancer patients and their loved ones through the challenging and difficult phases of diagnosis and treatment, encouraging each to adopt the same positive attitude that Lance Armstrong adopted in his own battle with cancer.

The Lance Armstrong Foundation is a registered 501(c)(3) nonprofit organization located in Austin, Texas. For more information or to make a tax-deductible contribution, please visit our website at www.laf.org. You may also reach us by mail at P.O. Box 161150, Austin, Texas 78716-1150, by phone at 512-236-8820, or by fax at 512-236-8482.

INDEX